Water Da

web site
www.waterdanceonline.com
Your anatomy is not your destiny.

Water Dance

WATER FITNESS
for
MIND,
BODY,
and
SOUL

Cooley — I know it is hard to get a mermadame to go from horizontal to vertical but please give it a try!

JULIANA LARSON

Juliana Larson

Paper Chase Press
New Orleans, LA

(I hope you & d can get Joan IN the water!)

Paper Chase Press books may be purchased for educational, business or sales promotional use. For information, please write: Special Markets Department, Paper Chase Press, 5721 Magazine Street, Suite 152, New Orleans, LA 70115.

FIRST EDITION

ISBN: 1-879706-79-2
LC: 98-068495

Cover photo: © David Madison, 1998

This book is dedicated to all those people young and old who want to make a meaningful change in their lives and to share their success with others.

I have many people to thank who have facilitated the process of writing this book.

My family has been supportive in every way. My main merman Lynn has been a huge part of this adventure and at my side no matter how deep the water. I could not have done it without him throwing me a rescue tube many times.

I owe a great deal to the Mermadame Society. It has been challenging to remain the president while surrounded by so many special women. Original members Gwen Garrett, Sylvia Baker, Alison Osinski, Ruth Meyer and Ann Cole have made the office a joyful learning and growing experience. Bruce Becker is an honorary member and true merman because of his strong commitment to each of us and to our mission. I believe what we have done together to perpetuate the belief in water and its healing properties will have a rippling effect.

I have learned from every person I have worked with in my career as a hydrotherapist and loved every minute of it. Every day I go to work at Sheldon Pool I am privileged to watch the thoughtfulness and courage in this world from its patrons and staff.

My book club has believed in me and supported this project from the beginning. I am thankful for their encouragement and positive energy.

I appreciate Werner and Lyle who believe in my work and took a big chance on me. With the help of Jennifer putting it all together, I will be able to get the word out to more people. Let's get wet in the process of becoming more of what we can be!

Contents

INTRODUCTION

Water is an absolute. Much like change, it is no longer an option, but a constant. Water creates, nurtures and maintains life. Water is energizing and healing. It is my mission to share with you the source of my energy and health, which is the wisdom I have learned from years of being in the water. I know you are looking for a new approach and you are open and ready to be part of something that will truly make a difference in your life.

On my 40th birthday, I was given a silver box tied with a black ribbon. Inside was a gift certificate for an astrology reading. Now I believe that miracles happen, but as a child I had gone to a real gypsy fortuneteller at the fairgrounds, and was not impressed. But I did go and with no more knowledge than my birthday, birthplace and time of birth, she started out: "It appears you need to be around water." Well, it is true and has been true most of my life.

In most ways I was an ordinary kid. I went to Camp Sumatanga, sold Krispy Kream Donuts as fund raisers on Saturday mornings, wore Weejuns, watched scary movies, drank Rebel Yell, loved Motown and synchronized swimming. I was never a beauty queen with my bowed, lanky legs, big hips, crooked teeth, freckles and naturally curly hair. What I did have was a mother who gave me great gifts. She gave me courage and kindness and a belief in myself. After my father walked out on her, she drew herself together, despite the frowns of society and supported me in whatever way she had to, setting aside the obstacle of pride.

Right when you need it life sometimes gives you just what you need. After a weak freshman year at a state college, I met my first "Shero" (not hero), the person who opened my brain as well as my soul. Her name was Dr. Rhoda Wharry. She was the most influential person in my life, teaching me passion for learning and teaching. Teaching children and future teachers to be teachers was her gift. When she explained things, her words were so logical and practical that it made learning a joy. She wanted creativity, individuality and resourcefulness from me and she told me I had a gift and not to lose it. I worked for her for 2 years and learned a lifetime of skills that I still use every day.

Yes, a lot of what I did for her was water work. I taught recovery and forward motion in the pool. It wasn't often pretty but it was joyful to see such courage. I taught relaxation to children with cerebral palsy in the water, which taught me patience. We got wheelchair bound children vertical in the water with water wings on a hula-hoop (not the child) and elastic from the fabric store and made them feel like they were walking.

Pools were designed for healthy, motivated, fit people. I made the astute observation that they would always be motivated and the folks that needed me were the complete opposite.

Introduction

Give me the unconditioned and unmotivated any day. I love to be with them. Why? Because I am surrounded by courage and kindness daily. They need my "bounceback" ability and my constant assurance that following through can make a difference.

Later in my life, I was in a car accident and sustained a neck and shoulder injury. Between the constant pain and lack of energy, I lost everything that I had built up—my business, my strength, my focus. I did not want this lesson, but it would make me speak from my heart to patients who were on their last effort, having tried all other forms of physical therapy with little success. The accident taught me a little of what many people have to deal with in their healing process. It took me over a year to get my energy back and I could not have gotten my range of motion and strength back without water exercise.

Whether you are rehabilitating or just looking for some outer strength or inner fortitude, you are in the right place. I can put a sense of control back in your life after months or years of that control being lost. It is a skill I can teach you. I have been shown the tools for improving your physical fitness toolbox. These tools are inexpensive and at your disposal in your community for your day to day maintenance or a complete overhaul. Bring a buddy. Do not swim alone. Start a mermaid club. Meet for exercise and support at your home pool. Use the tools I will teach you to take care of yourself.

I'm not holding a bag of tricks. *You* are in charge of your success; I just have the tools. Water is a way to get you more in touch with yourself and I have a simple way to provide you with the energy that you need to do all you wanted to do with the rest of your life.

Chapter 1: Water for Fitness

Water. It permeates every aspect of our lives. It is the origin of all life, and our bodies remain 60% of this magical liquid. We depend on it for our very survival. We use water for many things. We drink it, wash with it, use it for recreation, and many times we take it for granted. But water can give us so much more. For centuries, people have used water to heal and condition the body. Water can effect changes — physical, emotional, mental and spiritual. It can relax or stimulate our emotions and our minds, as well as our bodies. Water can relieve pain, help heal wounds, and increase our resistance to illness. It can strengthen our circulatory, respiratory, and digestive systems. Water can bring us to a new and deeper understanding of who we are, and what we can accomplish.

There are times when there is so much that goes on in my life that the path to getting on my suit and into the water seems littered with obstacles. A whole assortment of distractions arise, everything from what I need to prepare for my next business meeting or budget planning session, to mundane cares like remembering to pick things up from the dry cleaner, and what I should make for dinner. But I know that I just need to get into the water and tune out these distractions. The water will help me. The water will invigorate and relax me at the same time. *Water is good it nurtures me. I am happy when I am in water.*

Once in the water I find myself going through my exercises, happily absorbed by my workout. I feel the water caress my body, my arms and legs as I move through it. I feel strong and confident. My breathing is steady and my mind is clear. But perhaps I happen to notice the clock on the wall. And then, the distractions start again. I realize I have been in the water for twenty minutes, and my sense of responsibility nags me about this or that commitment. My temptation is to stop and just get out of the pool. *There is a phone call I need to make. I could take a rest now.* But over time, I have learned to tune out these things no matter how strongly they may seek to keep me from the water.

Any busy person (and who is not busy these days?) knows what I mean. We know that we should exercise, and yet there are always other things to interfere with a regular workout. We are often faced with the challenge that exercise is just one more thing to do and get over with. We like to eat, but we want to look good and feel good. We are getting older, but we don't want age to hinder us in any way from an active life. So, we know we must exercise. Exercise not only requires physical effort it requires time, but time is a commodity that is in short supply for most of us.

The challenge is to tune everything out and focus on being in the water. Let this be a special time for your body, mind, and even your soul. This can be a time to meditate, to give yourself some room mentally and spiritually. This is a time to reconnect with your *self*. This is a time to focus on something other than everything else in your harried and distracted life. This is a time to provide some balance in your life.

Like anything worth having, there has to be some doing to get the thing worth having. The doing does require a certain amount of discipline, and that all precious commodity we call time. Yet, you can discover a side of you which you will come to enjoy and I'll bet you'll wonder why you had never done this before.

I learned to enjoy what I call the *water dance*, a dance that encompasses my joy of health, physical vitality, alertness of mind, and an invigorated spirit. The water dance is body, mind, and soul joined together as one harmonious, joyous movement. It is the dance and celebration of life.

TAKING THE PLUNGE FOR A BETTER LIFE

Many people already enjoy the benefits of working out in water. Traditionally, the majority of people who enjoy water for fitness put emphasis on swimming. And swimming certainly is a wonderful way to workout and keep fit. Many of us regularly lap swim, employing various strokes. Some of us enjoy snorkeling and diving to make the water workout more fun. But the swimming only approach to water fitness takes a limited advantage of one's time in the water. A water workout can and should be much more than just a physical experience. In fact, a water workout should be a mental and spiritual experience as well. To focus our mental, spiritual and physical effort together yields a better workout, and encourages us to keep our course and continue for a lifelong commitment. Such a commitment elevates your feelings about yourself and your well being.

Something Different

A water dancer is different than most fitness folks. The difference starts with a medium that everyone is familiar with, but has overlooked as a very good way to become fit in all aspects of life. Most fitness people will do some land based exercise because that's what everyone else is doing. After all, when was the last time you saw a fitness program on television which featured water fitness? Running, walking, aerobics, and bicycling are among the most common exercises. And these activities are excellent ways to become and stay fit. But it is time to try something a little different, and perhaps more rewarding in ways other than the physical.

Enhance Your Perspective

Learn to get in tune with yourself, to communicate with yourself. Listen to your body and your mind. The water will give back as much as you are able to put in. Tell yourself that you can do this and that you will become a physically,

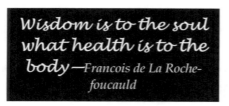

Wisdom is to the soul what health is to the body —*Francois de La Rochefoucauld*

mentally, and spiritually stronger person. People will sense this in you. Share the experience with someone you care about. Make this wonderful experience, water exercise, larger your own life. An attitude of confidence will build up from your experience as a water dancer.

Push Yourself

As a water dancer, you should expect more from a workout. As you workout in water, you should be aware that your body, mind and soul are connected, and that every part is affected by the other parts. The awareness of this can be exhilarating and very encouraging.

Our bodies are not simply sacks of chemicals responding to our environment. Our spirit enlivens our body and anything we do physically connects with our soul. But so many people just go about exercise ignoring mental benefits and the spiritual side of their lives. To just get through the exercise as just one more task in your routine should not be your goal. Instead, you can experience the fullness of connecting all parts of your being.

You begin your transformation as a water dancer by first crediting yourself for getting into the water and working out. This is a big step. Most people do not make that step, preferring instead to find excuses and do nothing. As you workout, you build your confidence in doing something regularly. You demonstrate discipline to yourself by doing something beneficial for yourself consistently, and regularly. In time, physically you also see and feel the difference in yourself. You gradually develop a leaner stronger figure, with more vigor and energy. And with the appropriate focus and decision to keep your mind free of other thoughts during your workout, you begin to develop the ability to have an uncluttered consciousness of the present. In other words, you become more aware. This awareness is a form of meditation.

UNCLUTTERED CONSCIOUSNESS

During meditation you are suppose to concentrate on a particular object or word, a mantra. The aim is to keep out all other thoughts. To achieve a clear and still mind. Now, the idea of meditation while working out may seem like a contradiction,

Pool Side

Working out in water can and should be both a physical and spiritual experience yielding an overall healthy body and mind. And this results in a much more buoyant attitude about self and life and people we come into contact with daily. Water fitness is very much a holistic experience. But it can be easy to let the daily routine of life interfere with the benefits that a regular program of water fitness can provide. I am always inspired when I consider the many benefits of water fitness:

PHYSICAL BENEFITS

- Dramatically improves cardiovascular fitness
- Strengthens and tones all muscle groups
- Relieves mental anxiety and distress
- Bonding with other people, making friendships
- Relieves or eliminates arthritis, back injuries, hypertension, Chronic pain, and a variety of other ailments
- Improves immune system to fend off disease
- Increases longevity
- Reduces bouts with depression

MIND & SOUL BENEFITS

- Anxiety and tension diminishes
- Insomnia is reduced
- Reduces number of headaches
- Helps create balance in your anxiety prone life
- Lowers blood pressure, reducing risk of heart ailments
- A keener awareness of self and the world

but it is not. Any accomplished athlete recognizes the value of focus. Meditation is a means to achieve focus.

Another way of looking at it is to think of meditation as a way to achieve a state of mind which keeps your thoughts situated in the present, the here and now of life. In doing this you are able to keep out the distracting, usually distressing things of every day life. It is easy when working out to let your mind hop around from thought to disconnected thought, oftentimes bombarding yourself with all sorts of wearisome, troubling, and anxious thoughts. You certainly don't clear your mind this way, but clutter it, and only add to the already existing strain.

Instead, you should seek to clear your mind. Filling it with the present and allowing yourself to blend mind, body, and soul as one entity. This idea of blending is the Zen Buddhist concept of oneness. Other proponents of meditation think of this as "mental centering." Some methods of meditation or centering include reflecting on prayers, poetry, and counting.

Getting Centered

You know you are centered when you can rest comfortably in the here and now. This is actually an empowering way to think. You will come away from this state refreshed and strong and relaxed. It is similar to having come out of a refreshing, and invigorating sleep. Water is marvelous because clear thinking and relaxation is much easier to achieve. Water is a very forgiving environment. In fact, the unique hydrostatic properties of water tend to relax the nerve endings of our skin. That's why you always feel just a little better after coming out of a pool, a nice long bath, or possibly a shower.

When you swim for fun, or splash around in the pool or at the beach with friends, you are not really experiencing the same benefit of a peace of mind work out in which you center yourself and focus on the here and now. Getting centered, being focused and allowing your mind to rest is only done when you are not distracted, even when the form of distraction is done in fun. Meditative exercise is a special time for yourself, to recharge yourself that can only be best achieved when you make time for it. It is a valuable investment into yourself.

> *The soul is born old but grows young. That is the comedy of life. And the body is born young and grows old. That is life's tragedy*
>
> *— Oscar Wilde*

And although you want a good workout and to experience the spiritual benefits, you don't want to allow yourself to get bored. Don't succumb to the "same old routine" rut. Make things interesting by pushing yourself a little longer, or try a more resistant workout. And try not to allow mental distractions to interfere with your efforts to get and stay centered.

Ultimately, your regular water workout can make a dramatic and wonderful change in your life. You learn to connect physically, mentally and spiritually, and you begin to look at life differently. You are more in tune with yourself and more balanced in your overall experience of life. You become a water dancer when you learn to enjoy life because of water, and your physical workout is just part of the way you get there.

Deep End

Throughout this book, I will be giving you instruction, encouragement, and inspiration for exercises, including physical routines along with the mental and spiritual side of things.

The overall aim of these Deep End sections is to provide practical, fun, and inspirational tips on achieving physical and spiritual balance. As for the practical exercises, we are going to get you in water and get moving. You will learn the basics of movement, of breathing, and even of nutrition. You will work hard to make things happen. While engaged in the practical exercises, you will work silently in an effort to cultivate our spiritual side. But to break things up, and make your workouts fun, you will do some guaranteed fun exercises with your pool buddies.

You will start out with 20 to 30 minute workouts, but eventually you will want to workout longer as your endurance and strength improves. Of course, in the beginning, if you need to make adjustments to your workout, perhaps make it a little shorter or vary the workout to keep things interesting, that's okay.

The important point is that you are in the water and your going to make an important change in your life. As you realize that you are getting stronger, which will be about 21 days into your routine, you *will* push yourself. And believe me, you will want to push yourself. It is a natural part of progress. You will discover how gratifying it is to change your life in this way. And you will see how it will effect other areas of your life. You will become so pleased with yourself that you will want to share your newfound joy with all your friends and family.

Chapter 2: Getting Into Water

Connie always says she should have been born a boy. Here is what she has to say of how water fitness became an important and integral part of her life.

"When I was growing up in order to play sports you had to be a boy, there was very little for girls to do. I don't recall that my parents ever told me or insinuated that I couldn't keep up because I was a girl. In fact, I was a tomboy and enjoyed it!

"Then I was in gymnastics all through high school and college. When that phase of my life was over I taught gymnastics at a recreation center and judged gymnastics. I never felt like there would be a time in my life that I would cease to flip, twirl or spin across the floor or on some piece of apparatus. I was hurt a couple of times, but I always healed and moved on.

"As my children grew up the activity level did too. When the kids played ball, I played ball. When they played soccer, I played soccer. Susan played volleyball and Debbie played basketball, and I was right there. We all learned to water and snow ski. Then we started whitewater rafting, and I wanted to row. And of course being from Eugene (the track capital of the US) I was a runner also. Physical activity was always part of our lives. I even coached cheerleading: high school cheerleading involves stunts and tumbling. It is so much like gymnastics, but you could cheat with spotters. Two of my teams took State Championships!

"Time has marched on, and in my fifties I have refused to let the body age. I haven't done real well physically holding back the process, but mentally I just don't give up very easily. And that is probably what got me into trouble.

"After I gave up the running because of the injuries, I discovered race walking. I am fairly competitive and really push hard. A group of my girl friends were walking in the world's largest relay walking race and asked if I would like to join them. A year earlier they won the event in the women's masters category. I wanted to join them and win with them in the next race. We did win that year, but I paid the price with a terrible hamstring injury.

"I spent the next 10 weeks in therapy and was then ready to start a strength building program. My doctor and physical therapist suggested I try deep-water aerobics for rehab. But I was very skeptical. Water is for fat older women not women like me. But the desire to move hard and fast made me go check it out. I continued the therapy and went to deep water two times a week. I learned that the harder the workout became, the stronger I became. Only then did I begin to respect the water and begin to rebuild my strength.

"Seldom in the past year have I missed one class. It is in my weekly routine. I need it. Vacations, pool shutdowns and the one time I forgot my suit, that's it. Now I have another minor injury and am rehabilitating again. Deep-water aerobics is not just rehab. Deep-water aerobics is also an incredible overall workout at whatever intensity level you desire.

"I do not believe, and neither does my therapist, that I would have been back on the road last summer like I was without the strength building from deep water. Yes, we did win again, the second time for me, and plan to step up our training for this coming summer again. Will deep water continue to be a part of that conditioning program? You bet. I am a convert. See you in the water!!!!"

CONVERTED SKEPTICS

Connie was like so many people who start off skeptical about working out in water. Is a water workout something you can seriously consider as a viable means to fitness? So many skeptics think water is too easy. That there is not enough resistance or that you cannot work up a sweat, or whatever. The most common complaint is that a water workout is not demanding enough. Most people perceive that an effective workout requires that we punish ourselves into fitness. You have heard the adage: "No pain, no gain." Well, the fact is that an effective water workout, if done properly, can make you very fit. But, of course, like anything else, you must keep at it.

With water fitness you can apply the general, all-purpose fitness guide devised by the U.S. Surgeon General. In short, the guide stipulates that a moderate aerobic workout for about 20 to 30 minutes, at least three times a week is sufficient to fend all manner of disease and debilitating physical maladies, including heart disease, hypertension, diabetes, various cancers, and osteoporosis.

But unlike land based exercise, with water fitness you don't have the physical stress, such as the bone and ligament jarring effects while running, or even walking. Water, as I mentioned earlier, is a very forgiving medium, and at the same time, can be very demanding. The fact is water is 12 to 17 times more resistant than air (depending on how you move through the water). So you are forced to work at least 12 times harder to achieve anything in water. And as you increase the resistance, intensity and duration of your water workout you will get stronger, leaner, and you will experience emotional and mental -balance.

Water fitness, like all aerobic exercise, can provide a balance of physical, emotional, mental, and even spiritual balance. Moreover, a water fitness program can provide these benefits virtually injury free unlike land-based aerobic exercise.

> *Iron rusts from disuse, stagnant water loses its purity and in cold weather becomes frozen; so does inaction sap the vigors of the mind*
> — *Leonardo da Vinci*

Believe me when I tell you that this will result in a healthier, more vibrant life without the pain land-based exercise sometimes produces.

So, if you begin as a skeptic about the value of water fitness, just give it a try. And in 21 days, I guarantee you will no longer be a skeptic, but a convert.

GETTING STARTED

You may already be in the water, swimming, or perhaps you have already experimented with water fitness aerobics, or perhaps you haven't so much as put your toe in water for years. In all cases, I will introduce you to a complete, mind, body and soul workout in the water. For the not so beginners, you will learn to expand from where you are, but for everyone, you will learn to change your life with a commitment to the water dance.

Now, it is possible that you may not be entirely comfortable with every single exercise or type of instruction I provide, or any other instruction you may read in this book. That's okay. My method, or others described here, may not be entirely for you. In the end, you may derive from this book only what you want to apply in your own regular routine. We all have our unique style in life, and I wish to encourage that in you. But experiment with different things, try exercises and choose the ones more suited to you. If you are big on calculating calories, apply what you learn here. If you are more inclined towards variety and duration, verses intensity, so be it. I know that after you have read this book, you will know how to achieve whatever goals are important to you.

What Do You Need?

Many people believe that in order to begin a water fitness program that you need to know how to swim. That fact is that you do not need to know how to swim. Many people over the years who have participated in my water fitness classes were non-swimmers, or were certainly no more sophisticated than dog paddlers.

Many women are put off by the idea of water fitness because it requires a bathing suit and that their hair will get wet. However, there is nothing to worry about in both categories. First, most people who get started are not in the best of shape. Besides, in the water no one can see what you look like in your bathing suit. Furthermore, one thing I can say with certainty, people who work out in water together are very supportive. It is definitely a nurturing environment. This makes the whole experience comforting and fun. As for wet hair, there is no need to worry about wet hair, since you do not have to put your head under the water at any time in order to fully benefit from a water workout.

The only real requirement for a regular water workout is a pool (either your own, a friend's, or a community pool such as the YMCA, high school, college, etc.), a bathing suit, and a Flotation belt. A towel, sandals or flip-flops may also come in handy (see more details on your pool bag a little later in this chapter).

Flotation belt? Yes, this is a special belt, usually made of a lightweight rubber foam material designed to be wrapped around your waist, enabling you to float in deep water up to your neck. The belt makes it possible for you to exercise your entire body without having to worry about sinking or remaining afloat. The belt also prevents you from "bobbing" (going up and down). Elsewhere in this chapter I provide photos and illustrations of one of the better flotation belts you should use.

These days, with the growing popularity of flotation belts, you may find a community pool or water fitness class that provides flotation belts. You can use those, but eventually you may want to have your own belt. This comes in handy when you are travelling or not able to get to your usual community pool or class.

Where?

Having your own pool is a nice amenity. According to the National Spa & Swimming Pool Institute, there are about 8 million spas, above ground, and in ground pools in the US. And if you have one, take advantage of it. You certainly will have immediate access, and it makes the pool convenient. Nonetheless, I encourage even pool owners to include scheduling a class at a community pool at least once a week. The NSPI estimates about 350,000 commercial pools in the US. The advantage of a class is the camaraderie, encouragement, support, and professional instruction you receive at a community pool.

How Often?

How often you engage in your water fitness workout will depend largely on your circumstances. Time is always a concern. But I strongly urge that everyone commit themselves to at least 3 or 4 times per week for no less than 30 minutes for each workout session. Of course, the more often you workout and the longer you workout, the faster and greater the results will be. But only you can decide for yourself what is good for you. And should you decide on the 6 or even 7 day a week plan, you will want to break up the workout with some variations, or you could easily get burned out and bored. But more on that later.

MAKE IT AEROBIC TO MAKE IT COUNT

You have probably heard it again and again from various exercise gurus: you must get your heart rate up in order to get fit. And they are right, even when you are in the water. It may be boring and not sound like much fun, but it is just an inherent fact when dealing with the human body.

The only way we can achieve cardiovascular fitness and become lean and fit is to engage in regular aerobic exercise, which means we must get our heart pumping. And for beginners, the question is always how hard should our heart pump? That's what we'll go over here.

Find Your Target Heart Range

Let me first define aerobic exercise with the following criteria:

- Aerobic exercise is steady and nonstop

- Aerobic exercise must last a minimum of 12 minutes in duration

- Aerobic exercise requires a comfortable pace

- Aerobic exercise must involve the muscles of the lower body

Also, for true aerobic fitness you must find your maximum heart range and workout between 65 to 80% of your maximum heart rate. You calculate your maximum heart rate by subtracting your age from the magical number 220. Whatever the answer, multiply that number by 60 percent. You may want to use a calculator to get this answer. Don't forget this number. It represents the lower end of your target heart range. Then multiply the answer by 85 percent. The answer to this becomes the upper end of your target heart range. For example, if you are 50 year old, 220 – 50 = 170; 170 X 60% = 102. 102 is the lower target heart range. Using the same formula, 170 X 85% = 145. 145 is the upper target heart range.

The most accurate way to determine your heart rate is to take your pulse by resting two fingers on your wrist or on the side of your neck and count for 10 seconds. Use a watch with a sweeping hand to monitor the time. Whatever that number is, multiply it by six. The result is your heart rate. As long as you are approximately within 65 to 80% of your maximum heart range, you are experiencing a decent aerobic workout.

So, in the above example, if you sustain a heart rate between 105 to 145 for at least 12 minutes, you are aerobic. However, having gone through this I should point out that this approach may not apply in all cases of people reading this. In fact, it is likely that up to 40% of you cannot effectively apply the magic 220 subtract your age formula to determine your level of aerobic activity. There are some people who have hearts that just go faster than most people, or just slower than most people, or have to take heart drugs. What do you do if you fall into this category of oddballs? Use the not too scientific common sense approach called the "talk test."

As you work out, try talking. If you talk and you are able to talk in a halting breath, you are probably aerobic. However, if you try to talk and you are gasping for air, and tiring yourself, you are working too hard. In this case, if you work too hard, you are no longer aerobic, but anaerobic. And anaerobic is really not doing you any good. The point is that you are trying to workout at a comfortable, steady pace. Push yourself, but not too hard.

Getting Fit

No matter what your situation, you will eventually discover that as you get in better shape, you will have to work harder to reach your maximum heart rate. Why is this? As you get fit, your heart gets stronger. And as your heart gets stronger it does not have to work as hard to pump blood. This means your heart beats fewer beats per minute. To stay aerobic, you must work out harder and longer to get your heart rate up.

The nice thing about water fitness is that you are definitely using muscles in the lower part of your body to get your heart rate up. Your leg muscles are bigger than other muscles and require more effort to exercise them. Of course you are also using your arms. And the natural resistance of water increases the challenge for your entire body, which is not something you get on land.

If you are among those people who can use the maximum heart range as a means to determine your most efficient aerobic workout, you should study the chart below to help.

Maximum Heart Rates During Exercise

Age Max. Beats/min.	85% of max.	65% of max.
25	195	166	127
30	190	162	124
35	185	157	120
40	180	153	117
45	175	149	114
50	170	145	111
55	165	140	107
60	160	136	104
65+	150	128	98
70	140	120	92

If you are one of the "talk test" people, just note your heart rate when you are exerting yourself to the point of near exhaustion. This would be beyond the upper maximum heart rate. This upper level is not where you want to be during a workout.

Slow down a little and you will be closer to where you need to be for a good aerobic workout.

KEEP ON MOVING

You know what you need to do: you need to get started in a new aerobic workout program, and a water fitness program is one of the most beneficial, fun, and overall rewarding aerobic workout programs. By starting it and staying with it, you will soon discover how you will enhance all aspects of your life, from the physical, to the mental, and to the spiritual as well. Just give it 21 days of consistent effort, and I guarantee you will see a dramatic difference in your life. And the less you have done in the past, the more dramatic the results.

The problem so many people have when starting an aerobic exercise program is staying with it. It's like so many New Year resolutions: nobody keeps them. The challenge is to keep on moving, to keep doing it. The nice thing is that most people who have attended my water fitness classes over the years, feel so invigorated and just generally better, that they don't feel right even if they miss a day or two.   Besides, the friends they have made in the class would miss them.

The trick is to stay with it long enough to the point where the physical effort meets the mental and emotional calmness and spiritual alertness. When that Zen oneness of mind, body, and soul connection occurs, it is then that you no longer view your water workouts as merely a duty to burn calories and to move on to the next item on your list of things to do.

Yes, it takes discipline and self-control when it comes to bettering yourself physically, mentally, emotionally, and spiritually. But when it is something that you can learn to enjoy and can see how it affects areas outside of the pool, you will find it much easier to pursue regularly. And why not? It is quite literally an investment into your self. You will be pleased with yourself to get yourself to do something healthy, and regularly that effects all aspects of your life.

Moving One Step At A Time

Rome was not built in a day, as the saying goes. And the fact is that when you want to overhaul your life, it is not something that is going to happen overnight. You must take steps, one step at a time. Perhaps you already engage in water fitness of some sort, but you wish to explore the spiritual side of your workout. But it is a gradual process. You have to be receptive, open, and willing to experiment. Or suppose you have never exercised in your life. You are a little intimidated by the whole thing because you fear you will fail.

Just keep in mind that you can never achieve anything until you have made that first step, and all the many steps that must follow to get anywhere. The first step for anyone occurs when you have made a very specific goal. Then you go about the business of achieving that goal.

Pool Side

STUFF YOU NEED

Water fitness is really not a complicated activity as far as equipment goes. But there are some basic items you should have to make your workout effective and a pleasure.

Flotation Belt

As I mentioned earlier, a flotation belt is an important part of water fitness. The Aquajogger® makes a great flotation belt. Of course, having the Aquajogger® will be useless unless you know how to use it correctly.

When you first get your flotation belt, begin by holding the belt vertically, with the Aquajogger® logo to the right. Start with the buckle end (without the prongs) of the elastic belt, push the buckle down into the first slot and alternately thread it through. Make sure that the adjustable portion of the belt is face up, allowing you to pull on the elastic to tighten the belt.

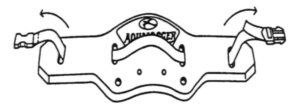

It's really important to get an accurate, snug fit in order to get the most out of your workout. To get a good fit, first remove any slack from the belt, position the non-adjustable end of the buckle (without the prongs) directly on the foam. Work all the extra length of the black elastic back through the slots of the belt over to the adjustable end.

Position the belt on your lower waist with the narrow "arms" of the belt just under your ribcage. Adjust the elastic belt until it is tight around your waist. The belt should be positioned across or just below your navel as shown.

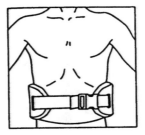

Adjust the strap until the belt feels almost "too tight." The tight fit feels more comfortable after you enter the water and helps prevent the belt from riding up or interfering with your movements during your workout.

You'll soon be so comfortable with your flotation belt you'll hardly notice it.

Various Resistance Gear

You can use resistance gear as a means to augment your workout, particularly as you advance in your fitness program. When you are strong enough and think you want to give additional resistance workout a try, there are basically three types of equipment you can use. You can use:

- water exercise dumbbells
- water exercise, zero-impact footwear
- webbed water fitness gloves.

Water exercise dumbbells are triangular in shape and are made of soft buoyant foam and padded grips. Excel Sports Science, Inc. has an excellent dumbbell called DeltaBells. To maximize resistance, you push the flat sides through the water. The faster you move the DeltaBells, the greater the resistance and intensity of your workout.

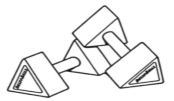

Water exercise footwear is designed to protect your feet from any impact, and to increase the level of intensity of your workout. Specifically, you can strengthen muscles, build endurance, and increase coordination. Excel Sports has the AquaRunners Footwear made of foam and a velcro strap to secure the footwear on your feet.

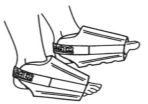

Water fitness gloves add intensity to upper body movements by increasing resistance and can be used with many of the exercises I recommend throughout this book. Aquajogger® makes a glove they call Webbed Pro. Changing the shape of your gloved hands, flexing or cupping them, or making them into a fist, varies resistance levels and can really add intensity for your arms during a workout.

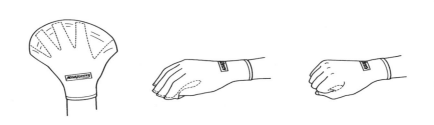

If you choose to use any resistance gear, remember to start slowly and build from there. Be gentle on yourself! Also keep the following things in mind:

- Always use correct posture. This is essential!
- Apply equal force in both directions of each movement to ensure muscle balance.
- Keep joints slightly flexed, not fully extended, to prevent injury.
- Keep equipment completely in (under) water. In-and-out-of-water moves adversely affect joints and muscles.

Stretch what you strengthen. When using resistive equipment, this is even more important than usual. Stretch at the end of your workout.

Pool Bag

You'll want a well thought out pool bag to make your time at the pool and in the dressing room as convenient and hassle free as possible. Pick a designated "pool bag". Any bag or tote lying around the house will do. Here are some things I recommend you keep in your bag.

- A beach size towel (not a small towel). You can use your towel for cover up to and from the pool. Temperatures in and out of the pool vary, and you want to stay warm to prevent illness. A short terrycloth robe may also be helpful.

- Non-breakable containers. These are good to transport soap, shampoo, and lotion, with your name on them. (If your names on them, they can always be retrieved from the lost and found!)

- Baking Soda. I have found using baking soda both at home and the pool useful in preventing dry skin. You can sprinkle it on a bath cloth, loofa or net scrubber. In the shower, mix it with water in a separate cup and pour it over you and your suit as you shower. Also put it in your bath at the pool or at home.

- Flip-flops, thongs, or water walking shoes. Pool decks are hard on tender feet; you also want to prevent athlete's foot.

- Bathing suit and bathing suit care. Use a suit with very little or no Lycra. Lycra does not wear well. See resource list for swimming suits. ALWAYS RINSE OUT YOUR SUIT BE-CAUSE THE CHLORINE MONSTER EATS SWIMMING SUITS!!! If there is not a swimsuit spinner at your pool, keep plastic bags in your pool bag to keep your wet suit from get-ting everything else wet. Or you can wrap your suit in your towel after and remember to take it out and hang it up to dry when you get home. Do not wash your suit in the washing machine.

- Small hair dryer, if you use one. Suggest at the pool's front desk that they keep a hair dryer for their patrons use. A dryer at the pool will mean you won't have to lug one around. You'll be pleasantly surprised how accommodating pools are!

- Witch hazel drops. If you are prone to swimmers ear, Witch Hazel prevents it.

- A padlock for "baskets" or change for pay-as-you-use lockers. Never leave valuables out in the open. You can also take your bag to the pool with you, or lock valuables in your car.

- Your own water fitness equipment, if you choose.

GETTING VERTICAL & OTHER BASICS

Before you jump into the water, there are a few things to learn. One of them (probably the most important in terms of exercise benefits and keeping your hair dry) is verticality, or what I call the art of remaining vertical.

When you get into the water, you may find your body's natural tendency is to slump or crunch over in the water in response to the buoyancy. To correct this, it is earlobes over shoulders, shoulders over hips.

Maintaining this verticality will not only promote better results from your water fitness, but you will not be subjected to back strain and your back, abdominal and surrounding muscles will strengthen accordingly.

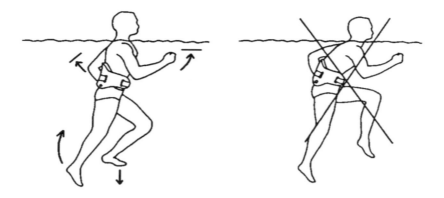

Breathing

I know we all think we know how to breathe as we exercise, but do we really? My experience is that without conscious effort, we often breathe shallowly or even hold our breath. In fact, studies have shown that most people use only a small portion of their lungs when they breathe. I want you to breathe more efficiently, which means learning to breathe from the bottom up. This will not only strengthen your lungs, but it will also raise your exercise endurance level.

Let's look at how we breathe. Our lungs are designed to use the air around us to deliver oxygen to and remove carbon dioxide from our bloodstream. Lungs don't take in and expel air (inhale and exhale) on their own because they do not have muscles. We use the muscles around the lungs — the abdominal and diaphragm muscles — to inhale and exhale. We inhale and space in the lungs increases (they "inflate"); we exhale and space decreases (they "deflate").

Your ability to control the diaphragm is less than your ability to control the ribcage and abdominals, but you can do it. One

44

way to increase control is to "push" rather than "blow" air out during the warm up and cool down periods of exercise (do not worry about breathing in – breathing in seems to be more of an instinctive, motor response). You want to exhale from the bottom up using your lower abdomen, lower back, and diaphragm muscles to "squeeze" the air up and out. Linda Farrow calls this technique "upside down breathing," which I think describes it well.

To practice breathing this way, stand with one hand at the top of your pubic bones, just below your belly button, and the other on your side, at the bottom of your ribcage. Just breathe as you normally do. Notice the movement of your abdomen and your ribcage. Now imagine that you inhale through the top of your head and clear down into the palm of your hand on your abdomen. You should notice your ribcage moving or "swinging" outward and your tummy "sticking out." Now, as you exhale, imagine that as your abdomen contracts, the air is pushed up and back out the top of your head. Notice the reverse movements of the ribcage and tummy. Make a "choo" sound through your teeth as you exhale and feel the contraction at the bottom of your abdominals.

Do you feel how integral your ribcage and abdominals are to your breath? Another benefit of training yourself to breathe from the bottom up is that you feel literally cleansed by each breath in and out. It's as if the air rushing in is clearing out the cobwebs and bringing fresh, new energy into your body and spirit. When you're workout gets hard and your brain wants to take the easy way out, concentrating on breathing the "choo" out through the teeth keeps the workout going strong.

SOUL FITNESS

As you pursue your goals and commit to a regular water workout, you will begin to exercise your mental and spiritual side. In part this means you will learn to center your thoughts by focusing only on the present and keeping out everything that interferes with the present. I will teach you ways to achieve this most effectively. One of the beautiful things about working out in water is that it is naturally calming to you physically, so the possibility of calming the mind and developing your spiritual side is just as natural.

There are some excellent books on the topic of mixing a physical workout with mental and spiritual renewal and development. One particularly good one was written several years ago by Al Huang, Chungliang, and Jerry Lynch, called *Thinking Body, Dancing Mind: Tao Sports for Extraordinary Performance in Athletics* (1992, Bantam). Another good author, medical doctor, and widely known advocate for combining physical, mental and spiritual is Deepak Chopra. His book, *Boundless Energy* (1995, Three Rivers Press) is especially good as it covers everything from nutrition to exercise, meditation, and reaching out to others. And then Joan Borysenko's excellent book, *Mind the Body, Mending the Mind* (1987, Bantam) really provides some useful insight into how our mental and spiritual side has a direct effect on our state physical health and fitness.

Deep End

GOALS

Set the goal. Setting a goal to achieve anything is a significant step in actually making something happen. Goals are something to aim for. They give you direction and when combined with visualizations, this makes the goal that much closer to reality. But a goal just in your head is not effective enough. Make it real by writing it down. For me writing things down makes the goal seem more real, more concrete. The other important thing to consider is where to write out your goal. Some people write out their goals on index cards and post them on the wall or on their mirror in the bathroom. This way, every morning and every evening just before bed, the goal is right there to be reaffirmed and re-motivating.

Of course, if you are like me, you may want to record your goal on a calendar. This is particularly ambitious because you set deadlines for yourself. Most people have trouble with deadlines. Each year, millions of people either wait for the last minute or ask for extensions to file their taxes. Cramming the night before an exam is another example of deadline dread. In any event, I may actually create a deadline for myself which dictates that by such and so a date I will reduce my waist line by so many inches.

At the very least, you are more apt to get closer to your goal than if you never set the goal in the first place. Be reasonable with yourself; set a goal that you know you have a good chance of achieving. If necessary, set smaller, achievable goals along the way. You might establish weekly or monthly goals so you are not overwhelmed by an ultimate goal. Then, go to work! Take action. Success can only be achieved with concerted action.

For many, perhaps most people, taking that first step is the scariest thing of all. It is a sign of commitment. You are, in effect, saying, "I have a goal, and I'm going for it." The next most difficult thing to achieve your goal is sticking with it. This is when the written goal can help. Keep reminding yourself of your goal to keep it alive. Avoid excuses that may prevent from achieving your goal. Make a conscious effort to decide that no matter what happens you have this goal to achieve.

The nice thing about goals that you share with others, such as in a water fitness class, is that people who have the same challenge surround you. This is good because your water fitness friends can help you stay on course. You help each other. They encourage and help build your confidence. The other nice thing about this is that before long you will see changes. In other words, there will be evidence that you are actually achieving your goal. This encouragement will keep you going.

I have heard many women complain to me that they just can't do it. But when they see other women doing it, they get charged up, and they learn to stick with it so they too can do it. And they do. Eventually they can't think of not staying with their commitment. That is the greatest reward of all. There is nothing more gratifying than creating a goal and achieving that goal. This makes the next goal so much easier.

Chapter 3: Womentoring

One of the wonderful things about women is our desire and our very *need* to help others. As a woman giving of your *self* is immensely gratifying. We feel a sense of fulfillment and achievement when others benefit from what we do. And because of the satisfaction giving yields, we tend to want to give even more. For some of us the giving becomes a compulsion. We even begin to feel guilty when somehow we think we are not giving enough. In reality, such giving can become practically unhealthy.

Of course, these days I see that more women are coming to the conclusion that they do too much for others. The result is legions of women who are beginning to resent this innate compulsion. Many women have ambivalent feelings about whether to continue giving and giving, or step back and give something to ourselves. Wouldn't it be nice to do something that can benefit ourselves and others at the same time?

Anne Wilson Schaef in her book, *Meditations For Women Who Do Too Much*, writes the following inspiring and encouraging words: "We women who do too much find the ending of an old year and the beginning of a new year to be a difficult time. There is always the temptation to try to 'tidy up' all our loose ends as the old year closes. We fall into the trap of believing that it is possible to get our entire life 'caught up' before starting a new year, and we are determined to do it. Also, there is the temptation to set up an elaborate set of resolutions for the coming year so that we can, at last, *get it right*. As workaholics, we tend to be very hard on ourselves: nothing less than perfection is enough. Hopefully, on this first day of the year, we will be able to remember that we are perfect just as we are."

WOMEN SELF-CARE

We as women must learn to care for ourselves. We deserve this, and we must recognize that it is just as important to nurture ourselves as it is to nurture others. Jennifer Louden, best-selling author of *The Woman's Comfort Book*, stresses the importance of self-nurturing: "Self-care is not selfish or self-indulgent. We cannot nurture others from a dry well. We need to take care of our own needs first, then we can give from our surplus, out of abundance. When we nurture others from a place of fullness, we feel renewed instead of taken advantage of. And they feel renewed too, instead of guilty. We have something precious to give others when we have been comforting and caring for ourselves, and building up self-love."

The water dance is one of those unique nurturing experiences that will never become a burden. Instead, it is a mutually nurturing experience for each person involved as you share together the transforming effects of water.

Womentoring

Mentoring is the ongoing act of guiding or teaching someone in certain aspects of life, whether it is in business, education, health, or even fitness. *Womentoring* is a special form of mentoring in which women mentor women on all levels of life including mind, body, and soul. Womentoring goes beyond just guiding or teaching; it is the nurturing of another person. And in its best form, womentoring is the mutual nurturing of two women who work together to better themselves with respect to their mind, body and soul.

This idea of womentoring is not just something someone invented and decided that there is this experience called womentoring. I have noticed that women naturally tend to nurture each other. What is unique is that water is in the picture. Water fitness affects all aspects of life in a way that nothing else does. There seems to be more support, more cooperation,

> *The greatest good you can do for another is not just to share your riches but to reveal to him his own*
> — Benjamin Disraeli

more concern, more encouragement, more affection, and just more fun than most other environments. This is what makes womentoring in water special. This is an experience unique to women, because this is a way of communicating that is alien to men. Men just don't operate this way.

Ethel's Story of Womentoring

Ethel is 83 years young and a wonderful example of how women help each other and learn to grow starting with their shared experience of water fitness. Ethel has always been a mover and a shaker, always active. Apart from an active life as a wife and mother, she has also been active in her community. In fact, she founded a non-profit organization called Driving Decisions for Seniors that helps seniors decide when it is time to let go of owning and driving a car. Her organization provides support, encouragement, and education to seniors in addressing this issue. Her program has been featured in the *New York Times* and on national television.

Ethel is clearly a unique woman who we can learn a lot from. She is very self-directed and independent, but it was not until after her husband had died that she started to make some significant changes in her life she knew she needed to make. But first she suffered through a yearlong grieving period. Then she made two priorities: getting into a smaller, less expensive living situation and improving her health with an exercise program.

Ethel had gained a lot of weight during her year of grieving and needed help right away. She knew exercise was critical to her health and she was going to do something about it. Rather than spend money for instruction she began to swim at her new apartment. But her commitment was not where it needed to be and the weather in the Pacific Northwest can make it tough to stay motivated. Added to this, her health (knees, hip and hands) started to limit her activities. Fortunately, Ethel's doctor insisted that she get her body (70 years old at the time) to a serious exercise program at least three days a week. This was the kick in the pants she finally needed to really make things happen.

"The water fitness class I started at the pool has been one of the most enriching situations I have ever gotten involved with. For 12 years I have consistently gone to class with the same instructor and many of the same people. Some of the best friendships I have ever formed have come from this class. Several people I have learned to 'deal with' have helped me grow in my tolerance and appreciation for differences.

"We have to know our limits and stay within those boundaries to be survivors. The same is true with water exercise. I have learned a lot about my body and mind while feeding my soul in these classes. Water exercise has been the renewing source for my body and my attitude every time in nearly all situations, and especially when I have a setback with health issues, finances, and losing love ones. I always return to the warmth of the water and what it does for my old body. I experience a wonderful sense of calm after an invigorating workout. I know that even at 83 the water fitness class challenges and encourages me to fight the aging process!

"I am also encouraged to return to water because of the caring people who consistently renew my spirit with their concern and compassion. I am compelled to give more of myself to them, and to others, even when I am not in the water. It is the nurturing you share with others during water exercise that has as much of an effect on my mind, body, and soul as the exercises themselves. This is what Juliana calls the womentoring part of water fitness. And this is one of the most important parts of water fitness I love."

Ethel's attitude and generosity has drawn many people to her, including a boyfriend about 20 years younger than her. I am very proud of my association with such a wonderful woman.

Ethel and many other like-minded women have discovered that one of the most beautiful things to experience is being in a pool full of women, working out, frolicking, chatting, and just generally enjoying each other's company, all the while improving our minds, bodies, and souls. Don't get me wrong, we all take our workouts very seriously. But the wonderful thing about being in water is that it can be both serious and fun at the same time. And being in water with women makes it a better experience all around.

There is an attitude that you adopt of helping yourself and helping others. A bond forms as women come together regularly in this way. They quickly share a spirit of oneness and become a sisterhood of mermaids.

SISTERHOOD

In our still predominantly patriarchal society, it is a useful and encouraging thing for women to uphold the sisterhood that we all share. As women we have that unique capacity to be in tune with other people. You can call it women's intuition, but the fact is we are just inherently sensitive to the feelings and needs of others. This is a blessing, not a curse. Instead of denying our inborn gift, or allowing it to virtually control our lives by overextending ourselves, we must learn to appreciate our sensitivity and take care to employ it with balance in mind.

Having girlfriends in our lives is a very important part of being a woman and we should cultivate our relationships with other women. I have seen time and time again how this has helped so many women in all areas of their lives, and it easily applies in the area of a regular exercise program.

Sheros

We all know about heros. And traditionally, most heros are men. But what about those important women heros, or as I call them, "she-ros"? I have many sheros who I know are worth honoring. Yes, I have sheros who have climbed mountains, and sheros who have started successful businesses, and sheros who have become influential politicians, but there are many unsung sheros. Ethel is one of my sheros. My mother is also one of my sheros. I respect and admire her strength of character, fortitude, and resourcefulness in raising me as a single mother after my father abandoned us years ago. And I have many other sheros, particularly my mermaid sheros.

Mia is another one of my sheros. Before her car accident during a downpour of rain in Seattle, Mia had been an active mother, school teacher, musician, and artist. She is now a quadriplegic who comes to the water to move all her limbs and her entire body in the only medium that allows her free, unimpeded movement. Her effort to improve herself is ongoing.

"For two months, I was without a manual wheelchair and the pool was closed, so I kind of regressed strength-wise. But the pool is open and I have my wheelchair back. I am now trying to build back up. I have been working out in the water with my helper near me kind of running interference. I still am unable to maintain (what do you call it? verticality?). I have no idea what aerobic pulse is for me, as it is all over the map and varies with my blood pressure. I am just pleased I am back in the water and getting stronger.

"Lately, I've noticed strength returning in my abdominal muscles, which I can move voluntarily now but still can't do any upper body moving, like sit-ups or preventing myself from falling back or forward. I felt strength starting to return in my pectoral muscles, which is very, very encouraging. My right pinky is also firing, but the hand cramping/curling is still so

55

predominant that I get discouraged. In spite of the hand disappointments, I actually operated my sewing machine, and got an extension on the foot pedal so I can run it with my elbow. The hammer dulcimer playing is coming along too - it ain't chromatic, so jazz and blues are rather limited, as are certain keys. But I am finding a way and learning its unique possibilities. Some things it is just gorgeous for. Next, I thought of harmonica. Why not?

"I find myself up against walls when I try to do art or writing of a personal nature. It has something to do with then-and-now comparisons; something to do with accessing that which proves painful. Fortunately, I have a counselor who makes it comfortable to explore these quadriplegic issues. I do anticipate a time when I will peruse these ideas I've been having. I try to trust the wisdom of the moment, when to push myself, when to just take care of business, when to retreat.

"I am starting to find other physically challenged people with these same health concerns, and swap ideas and remedies. Otherwise I remain the poster child for cross-discipline healing. But I'm particularly grateful for aqua-aerobics for giving me more strength, endurance, general conditioning, health, and return of neural connections and muscle function. I wish I could get to the pool more. But today is a good day."

Mia is my shero for a number of reasons, but one of them is her attitude, her willingness to go on despite the obvious limitations of her physical condition. I also admire her courage and willingness to try new things, whether it is a new workout routine or a new instrument like the harmonica. She is truly an inspiration.

Pool Side

SHARING WITH A FRIEND

There are a number of very good strengthening and stretching exercises you can do with one of your mermaid friends. For this pool side section I'm suggesting a couple of exercises you can do as part of your workout which is both physically beneficial and just fun to do with someone else.

Isometric Press

Start by facing your partner in either waist or chest deep water. Outstretch your hands and clasp your partner's hands at the wrist (left to right, right to left). You may have your palms up, while your partner has her palms down when you do this.

Now, at the count of three, you press up with your hands, while your partner presses down. This is a good isometric press that can strengthen your forearms, biceps, and shoulder muscles. You may want to count slowly to thirty before turning your palms in a different direction and then doing the exercise again. If you don't feel any discomfort, you may want to repeat this a couple of times, alternating your palm position each time.

Hamstring Stretch

Hamstrings, the muscles and ligaments that run along the back of your legs, should be strengthened to avoid injury and to improve your performance when exercising your legs. By stretching the hamstrings, you are also strengthening them. Here is a good exercise you can do with your water buddy to help each other doing what I call the Hamstring Stretch.

Start by facing each other in waist or chest deep water. Extend your arms forward, pressing your palms together (left to right,

right to left) while maintaining equal pressure. Now each of you bend your right knee and place your right foot in front of your body. Your heels should be firmly on the bottom of the pool. With each of you still applying pressure as you press your palms, you should both lean forward, continuing to apply equal pressure. Do this for about a count of 30 as you stretch your hamstring muscles. Reverse the stretch by placing the left foot forward. And do this for about a count of 30. You may want to repeat this one more time for each leg, but that should be sufficient for a given workout session.

Women & Water: Myth, Folklore, Tradition, etc.

The union of women and water is as old as humanity itself. We begin life in our mother's womb floating around in an orb of water. I have heard a man say that he has spent a lifetime trying to go back to the womb; often life does not seem as safe, warm, and buoyant out of it. Women have always been associated with new life. The various fertility goddesses such as Venus or Aphrodite are a reflection of man's veneration for woman as the source of life. Water likewise has been venerated because of its life-giving properties. All living things need water to survive. Humans cannot go without water in some form for more than three days or we perish. Water is the medium in which living cells thrive. Water is the world's solvent. The water cycle of vapor and rain is the world's natural washing, cleansing, and irrigation system. Two thirds of the surface of the earth is covered in water.

All ancient religions deified nature including all water sources. The Tigris, the Euphrates, and the Nile rivers were among the first sources of water to be venerated. This occurred particularly in those areas where early agri-communities de-pended heavily on water and the fertile sediment deposited by these rivers. Over time, many myths and legends developed around water.

In Greek mythology the god of the sea is Poseidon. Poseidon is represented as a bearded and majestic figure, holding a tri-dent, often accompanied by a dolphin. Poseidon was husband to the goddess Amphitrite, although he had many affairs with many nymphs of springs and fountains. The Romans identified Poseidon as Neptune, god of the sea.

Greek mythology also has several versions of singing nymphs or mermaids called Sirens. The more popular version of these myths are the daughters of the river god Achelous. These Sirens had such sweet voices that mariners who heard their songs were lured into grounding their boats on the rocks on which the nymphs sang. The Greek hero Odysseus was able to pass their island in safety because, following the advice of the sorceress Circe, he plugged the ears of his companions with wax and had himself firmly bound to the mast of the ship so that he could hear the songs without danger. Part of the legend sug-gests that when the Sirens were unable to draw Odysseus to-wards them, they threw themselves into the sea and perished.

In the Old Testament, there is the story of King David stroll-ing on his roof top balcony one day, inadvertently sighting Bathsheba, wife of Uriah the Hittite bathing. David admired her beauty and decided to seduce her while her husband was away. When his efforts to make Uriah seem responsible for the pater-nity of her child failed, David arranged for Uriah to be killed in battle. David then married Bathsheba, but the child died. Later, Bathsheba bore another son, Solomon, who succeeded David to the throne.

For hundreds of years in Japan, Geisha girls were skilled entertainers sponsored for life by wealthy men who employed them to sing, play instruments, dance, and assist bathing the men who attended mostly all male parties and social functions. Communal bathing and eating has always been a sign of acceptance and friendship in the Orient.

Native Americans engaged in a variety of rituals, most notably special bathing rituals. The bathing rituals, like so many rituals, often marked specific passages of maturity in a person's life. One important Native American bathing ritual was the sweat lodge. It had its origin in the polar regions and involved sitting in an enclosed hut, pouring water over heated stones to create a vapor bath. The ceremonial act of the sweat lodge was believed to wash away spiritual and physical impurities.

Swimming and just being in water lost its appeal during the Middle Ages (5th century to 15th century), when immersion in water was associated with the recurrent epidemic diseases such as the plague. People were literally afraid to go into water. During the late 19th century, amateur swimming clubs started to become popular in the United States and Britain. In the United States, colleges and universities such as Yale, Indiana University, and the University of Southern California also played an important role in spreading interest in swimming and being in water.

As Americans grew prosperous and increasingly open to swimming, along with improved pool building technology, more swimming pools began to spring up everywhere. Of course, the idea of water fitness at that time was still in the future. But interest in swimming, particularly competitive swimming, increased. And out of this interest, a number of remarkable swimmers made their mark, including some very talented women swimmers.

One of the first synchronized swimmers (originally called water ballet) was Eleanor Holm. At eighteen, she was one of the youngest American female swimmers at the 1932 Olympics to win a gold medal in the 100-meter backstroke. Eleanor Holm was a feisty, competitive young woman with a very independent spirit. Before winning her gold medal, she set several world records for the backstroke and placed fifth in the 1928 Olympics when she was only 14. Always eager for an adventure, she welcomed the opportunity to sing in nightclubs, eventually marrying an American entertainer and bandleader, Art Jarrett.

Eleanor's worldwide recognition as a swimmer and her interest in entertainment led to a brief career in movies (her most notable role was in *Tarzan's Revenge*). At about the same time, she began choreographing and performing as a synchronized swimmer. She was literally a pioneer in this early form of water fitness. In 1966, Eleanor Holm was elected to the International Swimming Hall of Fame.From its beginnings, despite its grace and elegance, synchronized swimming has been considered a very demanding and competitive water sport. All movements are choreographed and set to music.

Synchronized swimming requires overall body strength, agility, grace, timing, and musical interpretation. Much of the appeal of the sport is found in the use of music to demonstrate the athletes' skills, techniques, and creativity. There are three competitive synchronized swimming events that are generally recognized: solo, duet, and team (consisting of eight swimmers). Synchronized swimmers also compete in three categories: figures, technical routine, and free routine.

The first synchronized swimming competition in the United States occurred between Wright Junior College and the Chicago Teacher's College in 1939. In 1955, synchronized swimming became a competitive event in the Pan American Games in Mexico City. It was not until 1984 that solo and duet synchronized swimming events debuted at the Los Angeles Olympic Games. Americans won both events. Tracie Ruiz won the solo gold medal.

In the 1940s, movie starlet Esther Williams, dubbed "Hollywood's Mermaid," dazzled moviegoers with her skillful underwater scenes in a series of escapist musical comedies such as "Dangerous When Wet." Williams was a skilled synchronized swimmer. It is interesting to note that years later, after retiring from the screen, Esther Williams invested in various businesses including a successful swimming pool business called Esther Williams Swimming Pools.

In recent years, water has been getting more and more attention, and this is good news for we water dancers and mermaids. The more attention, the more likely people will be open to trying water fitness to change their lives. I have noticed that we tend to do things that people we admire like to do. In a recent magazine article, I was encouraged to learn that water fitness is becoming a part of the regular workout regimen for a number of stars and starlets like Sharon Stone and Winona Ryder. To me, it seems ironic that even though the majority of Americans are overweight and under exercised, we insist that the folks that entertain us on the screen look trim and beautiful. But maybe Americans need a little inspiration from people like these to get us motivated.

Women: Doing Something Worthwhile

As women we should celebrate our identity as life-givers and givers of ourselves to others. As we go about sharing with each other in the water, doing some of these exercises I recommend, we can take a moment to reflect on the significance of our place in the world, and be thankful for what we have and for what we can give.

Your experience as a water dancer will more than likely go beyond the pool. In the water, you nurture yourself and at the same time you nurture your relationship with other women. But you will also notice how your new invigorated self and enhanced attitude has a positive effect on people you encounter away from the pool environment. It's amazing how calm you can feel in your attitude and in how you conduct yourself just because of your regular workout. The balance you achieve through working out in water actually makes it easier to deal with the challenges that bombard you in your work-a-day world. It makes it easier to extend yourself towards others, to perform those random acts of kindness that we come to value in this not altogether kind world.

> *Shared joy is a double joy; shared sorrow is half a sorrow.*
> – *Swedish proverb*

I find that living to nurture yourself and then to nurture others gives life meaning. We all want a sense of purpose. We all want to believe that our lives have some meaning. We all want to believe that we are worthwhile. This is what gives you hope. There is no normal, healthy person alive who does not have hope and who does not want to think that their life has some purpose or meaning. We are not all just meant to inhabit the earth to consume its resources and propagate ourselves. There must be more

63

to life. I believe the more to life part is the perfecting of yourself and the giving of yourself. And the perfecting of yourself requires going within, while the giving of yourself is to go out.

Deep End

MERMADAMS UNITE!!
A history of The Mermadam Society

A number of years ago, I co-founded an organization called The Mermadam Society. This organization began as a professional and educational support group for women who are professional water fitness instructors/trainers. We encourage women in this field to hang in there and to not feel alone. All the members feel an important camaraderie, supporting each other in the work that we all know has life changing potential for many, many people. Everyone needs encouragement and support; it's a natural part of being human. By supporting each other, we know that we can be all the more encouraging and supportive of people who come to our classes. We are all committed to making dramatic changes in the lives of people who come to us. It is that which makes our lives worthwhile.

Through my association with my comrades in the water fitness world, I learned a great deal and developed some wonderful, life-long relationships. This is how I learned that womentoring is an important part of the water fitness programs I conduct.

Overall, I am blessed to have been around such wise women, true womentors, those who have healing ways with others. I continue to seek them out. I have been influenced by the way they teach and womentor. I have become one with them and want to share the respect and joy I have learned from being with them.

Everything is interrelated and we need each other to make life work. These are women who can access that place that creativity comes from. They teach through the five senses. They want to explore and experience all avenues when learning a concept. They know they are on the right path, but are open to inquiries and may improve a point or look at it with a new perspective. They are independent and are true leaders, seeking to work closely with anyone who is open. They are strong and work at being strong, but don't overindulge in anything. They are logical, but believe magic happens.

And magic can happen. I know. I have seen people's lives literally change because of their willingness to allow the water to filter through their mind, body, and soul.

JOIN A MERMAID CLUB
Women everywhere should join together in groups

You do not have to be a professional instructor to benefit from gathering with other women with the common interest of water fitness. And although I advocate that everyone interested in a regular water fitness program take a class at a local public pool, this may still not be your thing. Just know that that is okay. There are some very good alternatives. One good alternative is to form your own mermaid club.

A mermaid club requires that at least one or (preferably) two or more of its members own or have access to a private pool. The members need to agree on days and times to get together each week to maintain a regular water fitness workout program. The key to a successful mermaid club is making your workout program a regular thing. This is why access to more than one pool is important. You never know if a given member with a pool may be available consistently for every workout. It would not be fair to the others of the club if they are not able to workout regularly because the pool owner is not able to make a workout appointment for whatever reason.

Another reason a mermaid club can be a good thing for its members is that the group can become very close. This can be a very wonderful time for women to get together and cultivate relationships along with taking care of themselves physically and spiritually. Of course, some members may want to combine a regular workout with the club and include a class at a public pool for good measure. There is certainly nothing wrong with that. Do whatever is best for you and your circumstances.

Chapter 4:
Visualizing Aqua Fitness

Being fit is no longer just a way to reduce your waistline or to achieve a smaller dress size. In other words, it is no longer just a way to change your physical image. Instead, being fit encompasses everything about you: the way you think, your emotions, your attitude, and your spirit. This is nothing new, it is just that this approach to fitness is becoming more widely accepted. In the past, what was considered somewhat "out there" is now acknowledged as legitimate. There was a time when the concept of "mind over matter" was scoffed at by the scientific community. Such practices as hypnotherapy, accupressure/puncture, positive thinking, visualization, affirmations, and various forms of meditation were simply ignored as a means to health and fitness. But researchers have proven that all these holistic approaches to health and fitness are not only viable, but may be critical to good health and longevity.

BEING POSITIVE

Just having a positive attitude alone seems to be sufficient to abate and possibly heal a variety of ailments, everything from anxiety to heart disease and cancer. The term which applies when addressing mind over your body is psychoneuroimmunology. This term, defined simply, is the study of how our minds affect our nervous and immune systems. Our bodies are marvelously complex machines, and we are very capable of dealing with just about anything this world may impose. We can live comfortably, happily and healthfully in this world as long as we obey certain basic principles to ensure harmony in our lives. We have all heard the routine: balanced diet, plenty of exercise, a good night's sleep, and so forth. And if we follow these basic principles we will feel better, look better, be happier, and live longer. The funny thing is, we all have heard these things, but somehow can't adopt them. We eat too much fat, rarely exercise, are insomniacs, hate our jobs, and are constantly stressed or worrying about something.

I am definitely a proponent of psychoneuroimmunology. And I think everything begins in your mind. Unless you get things straight in your head, nothing is going to work in any other aspect of your life. If you don't have the right attitude you will not be disciplined or educate yourself about eating the right food, you will not exercise, you will ignore the warnings about smoking and drinking, you will view life in an unhealthy way, and so on. The lesson here is that you cannot separate mind from body.

Mind Power

Your state of mind actually influences and produces very specific chemicals in your body. Positive, loving thoughts release neuropeptides called interleukin and interferon, which have a healing effect on the body. In contrast, anxious thoughts or worry release cortisone and adrenaline, which tend to suppress the immune system. You can see this when you are both anxious and sick to your stomach. When you have peaceful or restful thoughts, your body responds by producing a chemical which functions like a muscle relaxer, such as Valium.

Your attitude and frame of mind also have a direct impact on the way you relate to other people. When you are anxious or preoccupied, people know this. If you are always negative or pessimistic, or have a sour attitude, people will not want to be around you. This is definitely not the way to "win friends and influence people" as Dale Carnegie would put it.

It is strange, but true that you can end up living in a vicious self destructive cycle of always being negative or pessimistic and end up with ulcers, chronic headaches, insomnia, or heart problems, which can only make you feel more awful and negative and pessimistic. It is as the saying goes, "You are what you think." And you treat others the way you think.

BEING GRATEFUL & BEING HEALTHY

I wake up to each morning grateful for another day. It may sound simple, and perhaps a little naïve, but it is the way I can feel good about myself and the world around me. Once you make a decision to live life happily, combined with the basics of caring for yourself, you can live happily and healthfully.

As a water dancer, I choose to make life a happy, healthful, sharing experience. This is what gives me an exuberance and gratefulness for life. This is what makes life meaningful to me.

Affirmations

Being happy, healthful and experiencing life to its fullest is something only you can make happen for yourself. Fortunately, there are some very practical steps you can take to help you make happiness and healthfulness a reality in your life.

> *More important than learning how to recall things is finding ways to forget things that are cluttering the mind*
> — *Eric Butterworth*

Begin by being aware that your words and thoughts have a dramatic effect on your life. Words have power. Words have the power make better, to encourage and nurture, but words also have the power to destroy. As you begin your water fitness routines and make water a part of your life, keep in your mind words to empower and encourage you. Getting fit in mind, body, and soul demands that we are encouraged, and that we draw on all sources of empowerment to attain our fitness goals and to maintain them.

It is a fact that actually saying certain empowering words aloud to yourself has a way of literally affecting your mind and your body. And affirmations are a way of impressing on your mind and body the right empowering words and feelings and thoughts.

For example, you can say aloud to yourself:
"I am strong and getting stronger!"

Just say this now to yourself and especially when you are in the water working out. Your mind will connect with your body. And because mentally you have made that statement, subconsciously you are making a commitment. Your conscious mind can decide what you want to say but your subconscious mind *records* what you say or think. What you put into your subconscious mind is what will affect your body and other aspects of your life automatically. When you affirm that you are getting stronger, you can actually feel that you are getting stronger.

I have some long distance running friends. And it never ceases to amaze me that anyone can run 5 or 10 or 15 miles with apparent comfort and ease. One of my running friends revealed to me that she simply affirms to herself before she runs that she is going to run a certain number of miles. By doing this, she empowers herself to run those miles.

When you work out, or really, when you choose to do anything, don't begin by thinking that you cannot do something. Instead, make an affirmation that you can and will do something. In the water you may say: "I will work out for 45 minutes today." And you will see that it will make it easier.

By starting with these simple affirmations, you can improve your attitude and build a foundation for yourself from which you will only grow stronger:
"I love myself just as I am."
"I am making myself a better person."
"I care about my mind, body, and soul."
"Water is good for me."

Of course, you can create your own affirmations of self- encouragement and nurturing. The point is to begin thinking positively as much as possible, and always seek to find words of empowerment. Hard as it might be to believe at first, you will actually feel the effect of positive affirmations.

Another form of affirmation is to simply put a smile on your face. Even when something happens to make you discouraged or angry, just decide that it is okay, and smile to yourself and everyone else. If you are able to put the situation in perspective and ask yourself, how important will this be in a year or two years, you can actually feel better almost immediately. Just try it!

Visualizations

Your subconscious mind comes into play in the area of visualization to help you achieve your goals and to generally experience a happier, healthier, and more meaningful life. Visualization is a way to train your subconscious mind to accept mental pictures as the reality you want in your life. You are probably reading this book because you want to improve your body by water workouts, but you also want to enhance all aspects of your life. Visualization can become an important part of the process as you create in your mind mental pictures of what specifically you want to achieve.

Let's consider your desire to get into better physical shape. Close your eyes and imagine, using mental pictures, what you will look like as your muscles get firmer, and you lose weight and feel stronger. You only need to do this for a few seconds, every day, perhaps during a quiet moment in the morning or before you go to bed, or possibly during the time you take for meditation.

If there are other areas in your life you want to improve, try to visualize these aspects of your life with mental pictures of change or improvement. Some people use visualization to picture their goals of the near future, such as the way things may occur during the course of the coming day or week.

Whatever it is you visualize, it is important that you do two things: have as clear and specific a mental picture as you can in your mind, and try to go about your life as though what you visualized has already happened. This means, if you visualize a more toned and sleeker body, start to carry yourself with the confidence that you are already toned and sleek.

By thinking a goal, visualizing that goal, and going about life as though you have already achieved that goal, the chances are that you will actually achieve that goal. It is like a self-fulfilling prophecy. How can this work? For those who use visualization as an integral part of their lives to succeed, they tend to make things happen to themselves, and draw things or people to themselves to make things happen with respect to their goals. Why do they do this? Because they know they have to take action and their subconscious minds are prepared for success. Consequently, they eventually succeed. Anyone can do this, and I encourage you to give it a try for your water fitness and other goals in your life.

Pool Side

TAKING ACTION

Set your goals, visualize and affirm those goals, and then take action. Taking action is important in all you seek to achieve. I find that keeping some form of record of my progress helps me keep going. This keeps me disciplined.

Calendars
I would get one of those big wall calendars with all the months and room to write something for each day of the year. You can buy such calendars at an Office Depot or some other office supply place. This way, you can write in your progress for each day, and check your progress at a glance.

Planners
An alternative to a wall calendar is something more all encompassing—a planner. In the planner you can have an individual sheet for each day to record your progress. You may even write, diary style, a brief note about the specific exercise you did, the duration, how you felt, your heart rate during your workout, and other particulars. Here is a sample planner entry:

March 11, 2020, Monday
Worked out in the water for about 40 minutes today. Felt a little sluggish for the first ten minutes, but everything went more smoothly after that.
Heart rate 120 bpm
Tried a new routine to build more strength in my arms.
Had a new person come to the pool, a real nice gal named Mary. She has had chronic back problems for years and finally wanted to give water a try. She said she had a great time working out today and will definitely return for the next workout.

Another nice thing about a planner is that you can look at it to see your progress over a year and see how you have improved and how your attitude has changed. A planner can be a very encouraging tool to check and maintain progress.

Charts

Some people are very graph oriented, and like to make charts of their progress. You could chart such things as your heart rate over time, the frequency and duration of certain exercise routines, good days versus average days, so on. Get creative if you want to do a chart.

You can either buy ruled graph paper to create charts or create charts on your computer with a variety of software packages. Again, you can find these things as Office Depot or some office supply place.

Scale Busters!

One thing you definitely do *not* need to check your fitness progress is a scale. As you work out aerobically, you will shed pounds of fat. But you will
also gain pounds of lean, dense muscle. The fact is that fat is lighter than muscle. And despite the fat you lose, you will build muscle and maintain a certain weight level. The good news is that you probably will not look or feel fat anymore. This basically makes weighing yourself on a scale irrelevant. The measure of weight loss and fitness progress is based more on how you look and feel in your clothes. Chances are, after the magical 21-day period has come and gone, you will look and feel significantly better.

MEDITATION

Meditation is essentially a means to improve concentration and to experience relaxation of the mind and body. But meditation can have important, far-reaching effects on your whole life.

By learning to concentrate and to relax you can immediately boost your health. For those who are prone to hypertension and heart problems, meditation is a strong prescription. Many heart specialists even recommend meditation (as a substitute for medication) to their patients to reduce and possibly eliminate hypertension.

Statistically, studies demonstrate that people who have practiced meditation for over five year were significantly healthier than people who do not meditate. People who meditate have 87 percent fewer heart problems, 55 percent fewer tumors, and 87 percent fewer nervous system problems. Other research indicates that meditation reduces the incidents of chronic pain, cancer, abdominal pain, chronic diarrhea, and ulcers.

To me, the most interesting aspect of meditation is the effect it has on your brain. As you meditate, your alpha brain waves, the waves associated with relaxation are initiated. This creates a restful alertness that tends to enhance your creativity, comprehension, and reaction time.

Beyond that, you become more aware of the spiritual side of your mind. Dr. Herbert Benson, bestselling author of *The Relaxation Response*, writes, "Meditation nourishes a feeling of connectedness to the Divine." The Divine, I assume, can be whatever you want to call it, God, Allah, Mother Mary, Jesus or your own personally meaningful divinity.

The significance to you as a water dancer is that meditation makes your water workout much more meaningful. You actually have a better workout physically, because you are combining the healthful benefits of meditation with the healthful benefits of being in water. Remember: water also contributes to easing hypertension and is a natural way to induce relaxation.

Meditate At Home

Just as I encourage cross training workouts (for example, a regular vigorous walking combined with a regular water workout), I also encourage what I call a cross training mental and spiritual workout through meditation at home and at the pool.

At home, you should set aside a private area in your home where you know you will not be disturbed. You should also decide on a time during the day when you may be less likely to be disturbed. Some people find a room, or a closet, or a corner of a room, which they designate as their sacred meditation area. You may have to unplug phones, turn off answering machines, alert other family members, and possibly keep pets away, to ensure you get the peace and time you need. But try to establish a special place and time for meditation. For some, morning or evening just before bed, are the best times for meditation. Decide what is best for you.

To begin, try to employ the so-called "concentration meditation" method. First, sit down in a chair or sit comfortably crossed legged on the floor. I don't recommend lying down, particularly if you are prone to falling asleep when you lie down. Rest your hands comfortably on your knees or on your lap. Now, close your eyes and focus your attention on your breathing. You can also focus on an object or a single sound. But focusing on your breath keeps things simple.

What you are going to try to do is to cut through all the mental static that is a constant distraction. You want to still your mind. You want to stop letting your mind drift aimlessly from one thought, feeling, smell, sound, memory, idea, or whatever, after another. You want to become calm and relaxed. By breathing slowly, deeply, and in a regular, continuous flow, your mind will become calm. Your breathing is the tool that enables you to change your state of mind.

Inhale and allow your breath to enter your abdomen; notice as the air fills you through the ribs and up to the chest. When you inhale, hold it in your chest for a count of three, which you say in your head: "One, two, three. Release the air slowly, exhaling from your chest downward in one, steady, silent breath. You should not allow your shoulders or back to slouch. If you breath in a cross legged sitting position, this enables you to breath more smoothly and easily. It is the process of focusing on your breathing, and keeping your back straight, that makes you more apt to concentrate and not allow your mind to drift to its distracting chatter.

So try inhaling and exhaling as described, correcting yourself when you notice that you become distracted. Refocus over and over as you concentrate on your breathing. Don t allow your mind to drift for long. Try to make your sessions about 10 to 15 minutes once a day. You may want to meditate a couple times a day or for longer periods later. Eventually, you will train your mind to focus, to concentrate. In time, over the course of days and weeks, as you continue to practice this simple form of meditation, you will notice how calm and keenly aware you become.

Meditating at home, in a quiet environment in which you are not moving is a good practice. But you can also meditate while working out, which we will explore next.

Meditate In Water

In water, during your workout, meditation can really be a rewarding experience. It is a very unique environment in which to meditate, especially as you are in neck-deep water and moving. I suggest you begin meditating in water the same way you would if you're meditating and walking on land. And as you walk in the water the natural movement encourages an alert awareness in your mind.

Begin by getting in the water. Remain suspended, moving only slightly to stay vertical. Think about your body and the sensation of being in the water. Then close your eyes, and focus on your breathing. Inhale and exhale calmly for a couple of minutes. Now open your eyes and calmly acquaint yourself with your environment. Be relaxed and begin "walking" slowly. Remain alert to the present. Center your thoughts on the now. Gently correct your mind from wandering. Focus on each "step" you make as you walk in the water.

Feel the water caress your arms and legs and body. If you wish, you can increase your pace, walking more vigorously, breathing a little harder as you go. If you are a beginner you may only want to walk 10 to 20 minutes. Eventually, you can extend your meditation water walking workout for 30 minutes or longer.

To help you in your meditation, you can try a number of self-encouraging power words, affirmations, or prayers to inspire your soul and encourage you to maintain your physical fitness level.

Deep End

POWER WORDS & MENTAL PICTURES
In an effort to have a physically, mentally and spiritually beneficial workout, you can use various power words, mantras, and affirmations to help you stay on track.

A <u>mantra</u> is Sanskrit for a sacred word or formula. For meditators, the main purpose of the mantra has traditionally been to keep out distractions and to help you focus, to get centered mentally and spiritually. This makes it possible for you to connect with your inner self or higher consciousness. Here are some mantras you can use as you inhale and exhale to keep a rhythm:

Ham sah: Sanskrit for the sound you make when you breathe through your mouth.
Om: Sanskrit and means *the beginning*.
Shalom: A Hebrew word which means *peace*.
At Peace
Be Calm
Relax
Trust God
Open

Because the words you use can actually affect your attitude and overall frame of mind, you should learn to use <u>power words</u>, or words that inspire, encourage, nurture, and make you better and stronger. Tony Robbins, self help guru and best-selling author of *Awake The Giant Within*, methodically describes how you can eliminate words you use which are dis-empowering to be replaced by words which are empowering. Here are a few power words you can repeat to yourself much in the same way you might apply a mantra as you meditate while working out.

I am:

Energized	**Hyped**
Unstoppable	**Great**
Unbelievably blessed	**Passionate**
Vibrant	**Compelled**
Strong	**Focused**

Much of the purpose for all these words is to keep you focused and motivated. Likewise, the use of <u>affirmations</u> in the form of phrases are important to help you set goals and to achieve them. Here are a few affirmations you can use, or you could consult a number of books on affirmations such as Shakti Gawain's book, *Creative Visualization*:

I love sharing myself with others.　　**Today is a good day!**
I love life!　　　　　　　　　　　**I am healthy & vibrant!**
I can do this!　　　　　　　　　　**I feel better than ever!**
I am getting stronger and more vibrant!

Another enjoyable and meaningful way to enhance your meditation and workout session is to make <u>prayers</u> or <u>meditations</u> a part of your life. Of course you can make your own prayers or meditations. As an alternative you can memorize and then reflect on a particular prayer or meditation. You can find prayers and meditations in a number of good books on these subjects, including *Psalms* or *Proverbs* in the good book itself, *The Bible*, or a book such as Anne Wilson Schaef's book, *Meditations For Women Who Do Too Much*. Here are some examples from Schaef's book:

There is something within me that knows more than I know. Trusting it can only result in healing.

Woman's work is always toward wholeness.

Owning ourselves is probably the richest gold mine any of us will ever possess.

<u>Poetry</u> is also another way to enhance you meditation practice as you workout. <u>Visualizations</u>, or mental pictures, can help in much the same way that words and phrases of words can inspire, nurture, and encourage.

Chapter 5: Water Fitness Habit

You already know that to really become committed to a regular routine like a fitness program, you must consistently participate for a magical period of at least 21 days. It is at that point that you will really begin to see and feel some progress in mind, body, and soul. Your achievements will make it that much easier to stay with your fitness program because you want to maintain and excel beyond what you have already achieved. For some reason, experts have found that it takes at least 21 days before something really becomes ingrained in your mind, body, and soul.

This is not to say that you won't immediately feel the relaxing and invigorating benefits of being in water. You will feel these benefits on the first day. However, to really feel your body begin to change in response to a regular aerobic workout, and to really feel the change in your attitude, to truly appreciate the enhanced awareness of focus from meditation exercise demands consistent, disciplined effort on your part for nearly a month.

EXCUSES, EXCUSES

I have encountered every possible excuse and form of skepticism about the benefits of regular exercise, let alone the benefits of water fitness. Time and again I have encountered people who say they just can't believe that water fitness will make much of a change for them. They have dieted in the past, and they have exercised at times in the past, and it has done nothing for them. But I challenge them. I tell them if they truly try for 21 days, water fitness will change their lives. Of course, I also point out something that Henry Ford once said, "There are those who say they can't, and there are those who say they can, and both are right."

Michelle gave water fitness a chance to change her life.

"I am a middle-aged woman diagnosed with diabetes two years ago. For years I had been obese, and have always been a care-giving person, often neglecting myself.

"My doctor sent me to an education center that teaches how to deal with the serious disease of diabetes. It was a rude awakening to look and learn about all the things that can go wrong with a diabetic body. It was difficult to assimilate all of it. One moment I was a fat woman who lacked the motivation to be healthy. Now I was a fat woman who had the motivation and needed to figure out what to do or face the very negative results of diabetes.

"The first reaction was denial. This, of course, ultimately doesn't work because facts are facts and diabetes doesn't just go away because you want it to. The next emotion I felt strongly was anger. This was so intense and I had no place to direct it. I felt betrayed by my body, my life and God. I had tried to do what was right and I had taken good care of those around me – but what about ME?

"I really had to learn how to take care of me. Juliana says: you have to care of yourself like the others you love and take care of all of you! You have to take care of mind, body, and soul.

"I created a food diary that has columns for grams of carbohydrates, fats, proteins and calories. I read about glucose and how it worked and why my body didn't seem to use insulin well. I read about exercise. None of it seemed easy. Information overload was in progress.

"I felt overwhelmed with all the changes I needed to make. I just needed to begin, but where? Exercise would take forever and going to classes with all those other people that do not have my weight problems did not motivate me. I put off exercise programs and went to my doctor about a new medication on the market to control and help me lose weight. I began the medication and it was like magic! I was losing weight, but some months later, because of side effects, the medication was removed from the market. It only took two to three months to undo all the good that I had done with the medication.

"The reality was that I had to get into an exercise program. Word of mouth helped me find Juliana's pool and her water exercise classes. I had heard of the program before but hated the idea of putting on a bathing suit.

"Resolutely putting aside my fears of what others thought, I began doing the class twice a week and after a year built up to a more difficult class three times a week. I felt better and I could exercise for the first time without hurting myself. Even then I knew three times a week was not enough; I had to get tougher on myself with diet and exercise. This time I had the confidence to take the steps needed.

"I began going five times a week to water fitness classes. Instead of dreading it, my mental attitude has considerably improved. I also have a feeling of belonging and being encouraged by regular people in the class. The wonderful staff is a huge benefit. The pool atmosphere makes me want to return and share my small steps toward my goals! My body feels more alive and healthier than it has in ten years. I can feel my body! Most importantly it helps me deal with my diabetes in helping to bring the glucose level down in my blood to a healthier level. The water workouts also help to increase my sluggish circulation and to take off some of this excess weight.

"As in all things the hardest part of this process was to get started. I found out my main problem and what to do to put control back into my life. This was just the philosophy I found in water fitness class. Be realistic! Be proud of the small changes I make and keep! I have changed my lifelong goal of losing weight to wanting to become a healthy person. In doing so the weight is coming off (I can see my tummy not my toes yet, but at least my breasts have gone down enough to see the next level!)

"I can kid again and enjoy myself rather than make losing weight my prime goal. Instead, my goal is to live an active and healthy life with my

> *It seems...as though the second half of a man's life is made up of nothing but the habits he has accumulated during the first half*
> — *Fyodor Dostoevsky*

family and friends. I no longer feel isolated and helpless. I have learned that you must put exercise in your life and keep it there.

That is the lifelong commitment. It is definitely for your mind, body, and soul."

If you are serious about better health, want to reverse the effects of aging, and to change all aspects of your life, now is the time to make a commitment to water fitness. Like Michele, you will know that it is the best decision of your life. The water just makes it easier to get started and to keep you going towards better health and fitness.

GETTING WET!

In Chapter 2, I introduced you to the basic requirements of getting started in a water fitness program. You need a pool to go to, have a flotation belt available, a pool bag to put all your pool stuff into, and don't forget your swimsuit! You should also find a buddy. At the very least, if you do not come equipped with your own buddy, find one at the pool. Most classes are filled with buddiers. In Chapter 2 I also provided some basics on being vertical and breathing, which you may have to reread. Now you are ready for the real thing.

I have developed a series of water workouts for you to make as a part of your water fitness regimen. The workouts are designed to progressively increase in difficulty, starting with the least difficult at level one, all the way to the most difficult at level 10. I will discuss intensity for each of these exercises and what intensity means to you physically and mentally.

The overall exercise session should include a period of stretching, warm up exercise, thermal warm up, followed by your main workout session, and ending with a period of "warming down." (Some people call it "cooling down," but *warming* has a friendlier sound and feeling to me.) Now, you can break up your routine by engaging in either endurance training or interval training during your main workout. You can also add a strength workout period during your main workout session.

Warm Up

To get warmed up do the following:

1. Enter the water.

2. Feel the water on your skin.

3. Establish verticality = vertical posture. Remember: Earlobes over shoulders, shoulders over hips. Neck tall. Pelvis slightly tilted to flatten your lower back. Relaxed knees, never locked. Collect your thoughts about this workout and make it the best you can do *today*.

4. Begin range of motion exercises which simply means walking back and forth in the pool, flexing, extending, and rotating all your joints (arms, hands, fingers, legs, feet, toes) or whatever your joints can do as you move through the water. Take slow steps and bring the knee up in a marching motion but never past hip height (90 degrees).

    Always remember it is not a biking motion it is a realistic walking/jogging motion. Use a pumping action with the arms. The fingertips are pointed in and the thumbs are up. This "cupping" action is pulling the water to your hip that makes you go forward as you walk or jog in the deep water.

Your warm up can be done in the shallow water or in the deep end with a flotation belt on. Repeat the range of motion exercises 3 to 6 times, add 6 to 8 times where muscle tightness is noticed. Once you have spent up to 3 minutes warming up, you are ready to do thermal warm up exercise.

Thermal Warmup

The pre-aerobic workout is what I call the thermal warm up. This is where you are starting to get your heart rate up, increasing your respiration, and making yourself mentally prepared for some real "sweating" should you continue to an aerobic main workout session. For beginners, that is, people who have never exercised, or who are just not quite at a very advanced fitness level, you may not get past the warm up and thermal warm up periods for a while. Eventually, as you get stronger and become more confident you will be ready to go on to the main workout session. The sooner you do this, the better. That's when some serious changes can happen.

1. The transition from the warm up period to the thermal warm up should be a continuous flow of movement. You do this by simply beginning a gentle walk or jog. Slow and easy look to the left - hold - look to the right- hold

2. Head forward shrug shoulders up and down as you breath (continue walking)

3. Roll your shoulders forward 3-4 times and repeat rotating backwards 6-8 times since this promotes correct posture. Gentle.

4. Hug yourself one arm on top then the other. Breathe as you open your arms to change putting the other one on top.

5. Use a row your boat motion. Reach, grab the oars and pull back. Blow your air out with each row. Squeeze in-between your shoulder blades each time as your elbows pull the oars back.

6. Continue walking and draw a figure 8 both arms at your side (by your hips), then out in front of you as you continue to walk.

7. Reach and pull yourself across the pool - open your fingers, grab the rope and pull your arms back. One and then the other.

8. Now flex the wrists and push the water away from you as you walk - shoulder height, and down, and return to the top.

9. Keep arms out front and flex and extend your hand at the wrist. Point up and down.

10. Bring your elbows to your waist. Stabilize them there and walk using the same arm same leg - like a mechanical robot doll. Think curl your elbows up and push the forearm down. Using the same arm at the same time with the same leg.

11. Continue walking or jogging if you are in the deep water.

12. **Tire Pumps or Sumo**

Use a breaststroke motion and open your stride to put your knees outwardly rotated. You will look like a sumo wrestler walking through blue jello or a jogging frog or a football player running through tires.

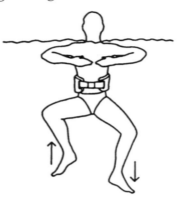

13. Bring your knees back in front of you and return to walking or jogging if you are in the deep water.

14. **Sit Kicks**

    Now *sit kick*. If you are in the shallow you will take a step, bring the knee up and extend the leg out. And return it down. It is up with the step, extend the lower leg and curl it in to the return. If you are in deep water you will stabilize in a sitting position. Do this as if you were in a chair. Your thighs never move. You are working your knees and ankles. Sit then kick out toe up. Return the lower leg in a curl under and point the toe down. Use a breaststroke motion or a paddle wheel motion with your arms to assist in the pull across the pool.

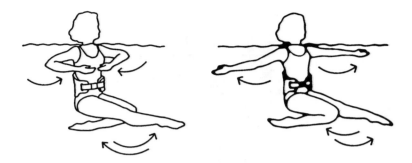

Repeat 10-12 repetitions. (Right then left always equals 1 rep.)

Then extend the arms straight out to your sides - pull them in front of you and clap and take them to the back as best you can and clap. Repeat.

15. **Cross-Country Ski**

Now begin a swinging motion front to back with your arms and take even bigger strides as if you were *cross-country ski-ing*. Plant those poles in the snow and slide past them. Swing out of the shoulder and swing out of the hip.

Repeat 10-12 repetitions. (Right then left always equals 1 rep.)

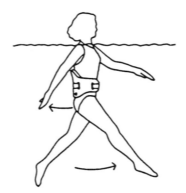

16. Scull your arms with a figure 8 motion and kick your self in the buns. Heels to buns -same heel same bun then change to heel to opposite bun one and then the other.

17. Return to walking or jogging if you are in the deep water.

18. **Aduction and abduction**
    If you are in shallow water, walk to the side. Step out, step together across the pool one way and then the other. If you are in deep water you will stabilize in one position and open your legs and close them. After several repetitions add the arms in the opposite way.

    As you do these you will look like the letter T then an A - when your arms are open your legs are closed. And when your legs are open your arms are at your sides. You will blow your air out as you pull your arms down to your sides. This decreases the bobbing action. The more control you have over your movements the less bobbing you will do. Remember we are not bobbers in the water like those floats on fishing lines. You will let the water support you but as you grow stronger and workout smarter you will "be catching the water" to add the strengthening component.

Main Workout Session

Once you have achieved at least moderate fitness (i.e., you can ride a bicycle for 20 minutes, or you can walk a mile in fifteen minutes or less and keep your breathing under control), you are ready to do the main workout session. Also keep in mind that you should work within your personal medical guidelines. I recommend you engage in the main workout session for 20 to 40 minutes of continuous aerobic activity.

A little while ago, I pointed out that you can also make your main workout session a little more interesting and challenging by engaging in either endurance training or interval training. There is also the option of strength training. However, I do not recommend this until you are in pretty good shape.

Endurance is achieved as you perform your exercises at a consistent pace, incorporating long body movements, while breathing comfortably. The primary benefits of endurance training are that you increase your cardiovascular endurance, body composition, and you burn fat efficiently.

Interval training involves alternating between moderate speeds and faster sprints. You also use smaller movements at a faster pace with rest intervals ranging from 30 seconds to 2 minutes. The primary benefits of interval training are increased aerobic capacity, muscular endurance, and fat burning.

For strength training, I brought up in Chapter 2 the benefits of using resistance equipment to increase overall strength. Apart from just moving faster through the water, which increases resistance, and opening your hands to increase resistance, you can use water fitness dumbbells, webbed water fitness gloves, and water fitness footwear. Again, the resistance is increased or lessened depending on the speed with which you move the equipment through the water. Generally, I recommend about 5 to 15 minutes of abdominal and/or arm exercises.

Intervals for Main Workout Session

As I indicated earlier, there are 10 levels (I call them Interval Training Levels) of your main aerobic workout session, starting from Level 1. And you should always strive to climb up. Even if your progress is small and gradual, the important thing is that you are climbing. Obviously, as you move up each level, the next time you come to the pool you can skip the level you can do easily and move on to the next one. Eventually you will reach Level 10. At Level 10 you will already realize that you can easily add other land-based activities you may have only dreamed of for many years. Just remember that it does not matter where you start, as long as you start.

Also, no matter how advanced you become in your fitness training, always begin and end each level workout with the warm-up - warm down range of motion exercise. And continue to emphasize any area of difficulty. For example, if you have an injured arm or shoulder perhaps as you are recovering from a car accident, place emphasis on that arm or shoulder to get it fully recovered and stronger. If you have chronic arthritis, you may want to emphasize extending and flexing the arm or hand or whatever that is giving you the most trouble. If you have a back injury, put emphasis on workouts that strengthens your abdominals. And so on.

When you begin your main workout session, start moderately and gradually work up to an exertion level within your target heart rate for 15-30 minutes according to your tolerance (reread Chapter 2 about target heart range). Take your heart rate in order to understand perceived exertion during your workout to know you are working at a challenging level. Levels 1 and 2 are fairly Easy (or light). Level 3 is Moderate and Levels 5 and over are equivalent to Hard.

You will notice that just maintaining a stabile posture performs abdominal strengthening exercises and specific strengthening exercises. Resist the water's buoyancy and control the movements. Use your breath to add to the co-contraction of the abdominal wall. You want to get the abdominal muscles to do 65% of the work, day to day and let your lower back take a break.

The advantages are many. Increased aerobic work capacity without joint stress in the lower extremities. The resistance provided by water exercise is greater than air and results in high caloric expenditures and heightened cardiovascular activity during the workout. The non-weight-bearing effect of water in reducing energy required for movement increases the ability to concentrate on correct posture, speed and breathing to increase intensity and perceived exertion. If you feel any pain stop the movement and return to a movement and pace that is pain free.

As you study the Interval Training Level tables below, you will note that for levels 1 to 2 there are three columns: Work, Recover, and Sets. From levels 3 on up, there is an additional column that indicates Perceived Exertion. For Work this is the most intense part of the training level. I suggest to keep the movement of this part simple for any level and only run or engage in the tire pump movements (see description and illustration above).

The Work column of a given level specifies the duration of a concentrated movement, followed by the recovery time, and the number of sets (times you should repeat that set). The Perceived Exertion column indicates how you should perceive your workout to be: Easy, Moderate, Hard, or Very Hard. During the Recover time, you should not stop, but continue some movement of your choice. I suggest you use the exercises I described above, including the cross-country ski, the sit kicks, and adduction and abduction exercises. You may use the exercises that you are confident doing, and spend the recovery time at lower perceived exertion and as a time to concentrate on your breathing.

Continue at the same level until you are pain and fatigue free more than three hours after the workout. Also determine your level of mental tolerance for the workout. If you feel confident and comfortable at a given level, then it is probably time to move on to the next level. You can repeat levels as tolerated.

INTERVAL LEVEL ONE

Perceived Exertion	Work (seconds)	Recover (seconds)	Sets
Easy	:10	:50	2
Moderate	:40	1:00	1
Hard	:30	1:30	2
Hard	:20	:40	3
Very hard	:05	:55	3
Easy	:10	:50	2

INTERVAL LEVEL TWO

Perceived Exertion	Work	Recover	Sets
Easy	:15	:45	2
Moderate	1:00	1:00	1
Hard	:45	1:15	2
Hard	:30	:30	4
Very hard	:10	:30	4
Easy	:15	:45	2

INTERVAL LEVEL THREE

Perceived Exertion	Work	Recover	Sets
Easy	:20	:40	2
Moderate	1:20	1:00	1
Hard	1:00	1:00	2
Hard	:35	:25	4
Very hard	:10	:50	4
Easy	:20	40	2

INTERVAL LEVEL FOUR

Perceived Exertion	Work	Recover	Sets
Easy	:25	:35	2
Moderate	1:40	1:00	1
Hard	1:15	:45	2
Hard	:40	1:20	4
Very hard	:15	:45	4
Easy	:25	:35	2

INTERVAL LEVEL FIVE

Perceived Exertion	Work	Recover	Sets
Easy	:30	:30	2
Moderate	2:00	1:00	1
Hard	1:30	:30	2
Hard	:45	1:15	4
Very hard	:15	:45	4
Easy	:30	:30	2

INTERVAL LEVEL SIX

Perceived Exertion	Work	Recover	Sets
Easy/Moderate	:35	:2	2
Moderate	2:20	1:00	1
Hard	1:40	:20	2
Hard	:50	:20	4
Very hard	:15	:45	4
Easy	:35	:25	2

INTERVAL LEVEL SEVEN

Perceived Exertion	Work	Recover	Sets
Easy/Moderate	:40	:20	2
Moderate	2:40	1:00	1
Hard	1:50	:30	2
Hard	:55	:30	4
Easy	:40	:20	2

INTERVAL LEVEL EIGHT

Perceived Exertion	Work	Recover	Sets
Moderate	:45	:15	2
Moderate	3:00	:30	1
Hard	2:00	:30	2
Hard	1:30	:30	4

| Moderate | :45 | :15 | 2 |

INTERVAL LEVEL NINE

Perceived Exertion	Work	Recover	Sets
Moderate	:50	:10	2
Moderate/Hard	3:20	:30	1
Hard	2:10	:50	2
Hard	1:05	:55	4
Very hard	:20	:40	4
Moderate	:50	:10	2

INTERVAL LEVEL TEN

Perceived Exertion	Work	Recover	Sets
Easy /Moderate	:55	:05	2
Moderate	3:40	:30	1
Hard	2:20	:30	2
Hard	1:10	:30	4
Very hard	:25	:35	4
Moderate	:55	:05	2

Warm Down

To warm down you should gradually decrease your speed and perform movements that emphasize those muscle groups worked during the main workout. The aim is to allow your heart rate to return to normal range, and to prepare the body to leave the water. You may choose to simply walk or jog gently, and performing gentle range of motion movements until your heart rate has calmed. This can take about 3 to 10 minutes.

CARDIO CHECKOUT

If you are experienced at working out and you are used to feeling different intensities as you work out, you will understand what the differences mean to your body.

It is easy to stroll, a little more effort to walk, and considerably more effort to power walk. A stroll, a walk, and a power walk represent three different levels of exertion or intensity. You need to develop the understanding of intensity and what feels right for you. The more you do it, the easier it will be.

The cardiovascular aspect of your workout is equally as important as the stretching and strengthening component of the workouts and must be included in your week. Going to the water includes each of these in a moderate to somewhat hard level.

One of the distinct advantages of working out in water, unlike any other environment is that you get a 3-dimensional workout for your muscles: top to bottom, front to back, and side to side. Monitoring your exercise intensity can be as simple as the talk test I described in Chapter 2, in which you check to see if you have enough breath control to talk while working out. Ask yourself: are you talking too much or singing? Then maybe your exercise routine is a bit too easy.

Add Intensity

Blow out your air when the going gets tough. Decrease the range of motion of the move - increase the speed. No bobbing! With every repetition, add intensity by forcing air out.

Reverse Aging

So much of the decrease in physical fitness and ability is attributed to the aging process when really it is just being inactive that increases the aging process. You are never too old to exercise or to start exercising! A balanced program of water and weights can slow and even reverse many of those common aging aggravations and disappointments.

Aerobic exercise improves the cardiovascular health of the heart, therefore decreasing your risk of a heart attack or stroke. In order to be aerobic you must engage in an activity that nudges your endurance and the muscles, bones, joints, the heart and lungs. These bodily systems become stronger and healthier under this strength training. Water fitness is ideal because in the water the "stress" on the joints is all but removed but the benefits to the systems remain. The fatigue factor is also negated because the water cools your body, leaving you with the energy to work out and not be drained from overheating.

Muscle and joint strengthening can be done at any age. Old muscles do respond to training by getting larger and of course stronger. You exert muscle power (no matter what level) against water and

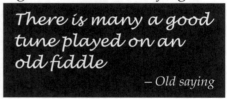

There is many a good tune played on an old fiddle

— Old saying

you learn that water can dish out as much as you can take! You are in charge of how strong you become. It will be very encouraging as you feel yourself gaining strength. Your activities of daily living will become a bit easier. You will notice that you have a better capacity for balance while walking on trails or doing housework. You are less fatigued while shopping or dodging retail challenged individuals. Your movements become more confident. You will notice being more physically

101

flexible, which along with balance will make you less suscepti-ble to a falling injury.

In the water you are working with cooperative movements that make you more capable of other challenges life gives you or challenges you choose to give yourself. People who exercise at pools often talk of how uplifted they feel after their water work-out. It is certainly because of the water and weight workout, but it is also the psychological benefit of exercising within a supportive environment.

DIET & NUTRITION

As you work out regularly in water, you will notice that your appetite will eventually come under control. Yes, this can hap-pen even if you have had a problem with food and your weight for years. Why? Aerobic exercise has an added benefit of mak-ing your appestat (your body's natural automatic appetite-control mechanism) effective. For many weight-challenged people, an appestat may sound like a myth. That is probably because years of overeating have rendered your appestat inop-erable, and controlling your appetite only results once you have stuffed yourself with food. You literally override the effective-ness of your appestat by simply continuing to eat even though your body is trying to tell you, "Enough, already!"

To help you with food, I want to spend a little time here on diet and nutrition. Diet and nutrition are also essential to the overall program when you are serious about making a lifestyle change that encompasses your mind, body, and soul.

Diets Don't Work!

First of all, unless you have been living under a rock for the past twenty years, you have probably already heard some diet guru proclaiming that diets do not work. Of course this is just the opposite to what diet experts had been saying for years earlier. For decades, once people realized that they were fat because of food, to them the obvious answer to being fat was to diet. All sorts of diets have come and gone over the years. I have heard of all protein diets, and liquid diets, the fruit and vegetable diet, the cabbage soup diet, the Scarsdale diet, and on and on. We know now that the answer to being fat is to stop eating fat and start exercising!

The exercise part is something we are addressing with the water fitness you incorporate into your life. Let's talk about the food you need in your diet. Get the word "diet" out of your vocabulary within the context of losing weight. Diet is the food you eat. And you are not trying to lose weight; you are trying to and shall lose fat.

You know what you should not eat. You should not eat practically all that junk you buy at fast food places, and everything loaded with 25% or more fat in calories per serving (cookies, cakes, doughnuts, french fries, ice cream, potato chips, bacon, etc., etc.). I recommend that you simply do not buy all the stuff you know you should not eat, and throw out the bad stuff from your house. This is not to say you can't have something wicked every once in a while. But at least make it scarce in your home because I guarantee that if you have it in your home, you will find it, and you will consume it.

I understand that getting rid of the fat food from your life is easier said than done, especially if you are a Southerner and lived with your grandmother as a child. This is particularly

103

challenging if you have been used to eating fat food for many years, perhaps decades. Our bodies become literally addicted to the fat. We crave it, yearn for it. The last thing we want to do is to stop eating it. But you know you need to so the best way to stop eating most of the fat is to keep as much of it out of your house as possible.

Keep It Simple

Since dieting does not work, and you still need to eat, what should you eat? The answer is so simple, you may find it difficult to accept. I say that because it seems that we are always looking for some magical solution.

The magical solution comes down to eating a balanced and varied selection of food from the four basic food groups that you probably remember from grade school. In case you forgot, the groups are: meats, dairy products, fruits and vegetables, breads and cereals.

When selecting food from each of these groups, keep the following simple rules in mind:

- Eat foods low in fat
- Eat foods low in sugar
- Eat foods high in fiber

Another simple rule to follow is that you should always try to eat food the closest to its natural state as possible. For example, try to eat whole grain breads versus highly refined white bread. Take a look at the label some time when you are shopping and you won't believe what can be in most brand name foods! Whole grain bread is closer to the natural state of wheat and yields vitamins and minerals removed from white bread through the refinement process. This makes it more desirable and more beneficial for your body. Eating organically produced food is good, but just keep in mind the fat calories as not all organic foods are low in fat.

Also, rather than a high calorie, low-fiber glass of orange juice, eat a lower calorie, high fiber orange or two in the morning. You will improve your digestion by eating 20-35 grams of fiber each day. People who are into juicing fruits and vegetables lose out on the benefits of the very important fiber and minerals contained in fruits and vegetables. Rather than juicing, just eat the fruit or vegetable without doing anything to it, although you might make a fruit salad or leafy salads with non-fat dressing, or simple stir fry dishes.

Of course there are some exceptions of foods which, even in their natural state, you should eat only occasionally. These are foods that are quite fattening, and you should just learn the most popular ones such as eggs, avocados, nuts and seeds of any kind, and olives. Butter cannot really be considered a food, but we don't need anyone to tell us that butter is not part of a well-balanced diet! We have been hearing that for years and know that while it is tempting, it is better to smear jam on than the greasy stuff.

Fat Versus Nutrition

We should always seek nutrients in our food. But this can be challenging, as there are foods that have a high nutrient content, but also have a high fat content. Red meat, for example, is nutritious because it is rich in protein and nutritious minerals. But red meat, like a thick steak, is also high in fat content. A healthier, leaner red meat alternative is wild game such as rabbit, deer, or quail. Better yet, you should consider skipping red meat altogether and eat protein rich, low-fat, high fiber beans. Pork is generally fatty, particularly bacon, although pigs are being raised these days to yield leaner meat. Chicken is lean as long as you remove the skin before cooking.

Milk has important nutrients no matter what the fat content. To me this means there is no reason to drink whole milk with a higher fat content when non-fat skim milk is just as nutritious. This applies to low-fat and non-fat cheeses, too. Of course, there are some cheeses that don't easily lend themselves to low-fat or non-fat products that taste like their full fat counterparts. You have to experiment with different products. Right now cottage cheese, part-skim mozzarella, American, and cheddar cheeses seem to be decent tasting with most of the fat and virtually none of the nutrients removed.

Ultimately, the most effective way to ensure that you are getting a sufficient combination of nutrients in your diet, while eating foods that are low-fat, low-sugar, and high fiber, is to strive for balance. And balance is achieved by selecting things from the four basic food groups. As a guide to determine how many items to select from each food group, try to select two items each from the meat group and the dairy product group, and four items each from the breads and cereals group and the fruits and vegetables group.

Fortunately, you have a couple of things going for you as a person engaged in regular aerobic activity. First, you will naturally burn fat because of your exercise. Second, your newly engaged appestat will help you curb your hunger. Your body will let you know when it is hungry. It is not a bad thing to snack or have several little meals throughout the day, just make sure that you follow the rules. Since you won't have junk around the house, and instead will have mostly healthful foods such as whole grained breads or fruits and vegetables, munch on those items.

Finally, while you don't want to accumulate tons of calories, fat grams or percentage of fat in the foods you eat is even more significant. Pay particular attention to the fat content of processed foods, or basically anything that comes in a package. If you need to burn more than 25 pounds of fat, consider eating foods no more than 10% fat, otherwise you can probably get trim or stay trim by eating foods with no more than 20 to 25% fat. Most packaging these days informs you about fat content, so read it. Generally, anything that is not packaged is probably fairly low in fat, sugar, and calories.

MAKE HEALTHFUL FOOD INTERESTING

One of the greatest challenges with eating low-fat, low-sugar, high fiber foods is that it is not as fun or satisfying to eat them like fat foods. Let's face it, fat filled foods are just more enjoyable. Eating cheese laden, juicy hamburgers and a sack full of fries is just sheer pleasure. And who wouldn't want to gorge themselves on a nice slice of pizza?

How do we make healthful foods more enjoyable? There are a variety of ways and I'll make a few suggestions here. Keep in mind, however, that what you need is a whole new attitude towards food. Be willing to educate yourself about food and then make the wisest choices. Your aim is to eat for health. By taking the balanced diet approach that I have outlined here, you will automatically lose fat. You will also be supplying your body with the right amount of nutrients to live a healthy, vibrant, longer life.

- Keeping a journal of calorie consumption is an eye open-ing experience. It is a good thing to start realizing how much and what we have been putting into our bodies.

- We are what we eat. It is our fuel to be able to work and play.

- Always share a dessert.

- Try eating small healthy meals throughout the day. Do not skip breakfast.

- Keep your portion size down of the food you eat. Think about it before you go back for seconds.

- You want to exercise to get more lean muscle mass. With more muscle power you have the potential to burn more calories.

Metabolism is the rate at which your body burns calories, and diet and exercise play an important role in that battle against adding weight as we age. We must keep our metabolism up and that takes effort. Your brain will always take the easy way out. You must resist the easy couch potato path. Walk instead of ride, eat more fish and legumes, cook from scratch , take a cooking class, stretch while watching T.V., grow your own small garden, drink more water, go to bed early and try a weight lift-ing program. A good book that I highly recommend is Daniel Kosich 's, *Get Real: Guide to Real-Life Weight Management.*

Sauces, Dressings, & Gravies Oh My!!

We humans have ingenious ways of taking otherwise healthy foods and turning them into health nightmares. We take vitamin and mineral rich greens and other vegetables and put them in salads laden with fat rich, heart threatening dressing. Or we take a healthy, nutritious baked potato and defile it with gobs of butter. We can't help it—it's in our nature to want things to be more interesting. So, here are a few simple suggestions on how you can find alternative sauces, dressings, and various toppings to make food palatable without ruining your health:

Butter substitutes: low-fat or non-fat sour cream, or cottage cheese or plain non-fat yogurt. Applesauce is good for baking.

Toppings: Jams and jellies are non-fat and good for toast, bagels, or whatever. As I indicated earlier, there are some decent low-fat and non-fat cheeses for pizza, sandwiches, etc.

Gravies & Sauces: Low-fat or non-fat soups like mushroom soup, tomato based sauces flavored with various seasoning.

There are a number of good books that have excellent recipes for low-fat or non-fat sauces, gravies, dips, deserts, salad dressings, and so on. Check out your local bookstore; there is usually a section filled with books for people who are looking to make a serious change in their eating and cooking habits.

Remember that just because you are adopting a new way to view food, this does not mean you can no longer enjoy eating. You can, you just have to find sensible alternatives.

Soul Food Recipes

I'm from the South, and we southerners love to eat. The trouble is that many favorite southern dishes are not exactly fat and calorie conscious. Fortunately, people with similar concerns about healthy eating have managed to create some very good healthful versions of some southern favorites. Here are some good recipes you may want to try.

Soul food - Take as needed for a comfort fix.

Cornbread – my Grandmother Mrs. Elna Cullom's recipe

Preheat oven to 400°

3/4 cup cornmeal	3/4 t baking powder
1/4 cup flour	3/8 t soda
1/2 t salt	1 big egg, beaten
2/3 cup buttermilk or sour milk*	

Oil a skillet or muffin pan and put in the oven while mixing the batter.

Sift all dry ingredients in mixing bowl. Mix egg with milk and lightly stir into dry mixture until just moistened. Pour immediately into hot skillet or muffin pan. Bake at 400 degrees about 20 minutes.

*(To make sour milk, add 1 T vinegar or lemon juice per cup of fresh milk.)

110

Things that go great with cornbread:

– Corn on the cob
– 1 peeled cucumber, tiny bit of onion and 1 tomato with just a tablespoon of mayonnaise.
– Beans and rice, but especially black-eyed peas! You can just open the can but I follow the directions on the dried peas package – you can use olive oil instead of chunk of pork.

Orange and Onion Tossed Salad – Mrs. Tom Thrasher

Salad:
2 cups bite size pieces of romaine lettuce
1 cup bite size pieces of chicory
1 cup bite size pieces of escarole
2 med. Oranges
1/4 cup purple onion rings, thinly sliced

Dressing:
1 clove garlic
¼ cup olive oil
2 T lemon juice
¼ t salt

1/4 t sugar
1/4 t dry mustard
1/4 t coarsely ground black pepper

Combine greens in a bowl. Peel oranges and cut into thin crosswise slices.

Arrange orange slices and onion rings over greens. Put in refrigerator.

Dressing: (Make 1 hour ahead if possible.) Dice garlic and put in oil. Add remaining ingredients and beat with a whisk. Pour over salad right before serving and toss. 6 servings.

Yancey County Cobbler
(~~~~Batter on the butter and the fruit on the top~~~~)
Preheat oven to 350°

1-2 T margarine	½ c sugar
1 c whole wheat flour	1 c low fat or skim milk
2 t baking powder	2 c fresh berries or apples

In oven, melt margarine in 9"x 9" square pan.
Mix flour, baking powder, and sugar. Add milk, mix. Pour mixture over melted butter in pan.
Pour fruit over batter, and just slightly stir.
Bake for 25 minutes or until golden brown crust surrounds the fruit. Enjoy with a small amount of milk!

Ambrosia
We have this for every special occasion. (My mother sends us pecans so we will have the right stuff.) It takes all of us cutting up the fruit but it's worth it!

Apples - one for every one, cut into bite size pieces
Oranges - one for every one, peeled and cut into bite size pieces
2 Cups red seedless grapes, cut in half
Juice of one 1 extra orange
Fresh coconut to taste
Chopped pecans to taste
Gently toss all ingredients together.
Serve in a beautiful glass bowl (from your grandmother)

Pool Side

Travelling can sometimes make it challenging to continue your exercise and diet program, the following tips can help.

TRAVEL TIPS

Whether you're travelling for a weekend jaunt or a two or three week vacation, you should:

- Call ahead to make sure the hotel has a pool. Find out if it is heated.
- Take your Aquajogger with you to workout in the pool at the hotel or campground.
- Use the stairs no matter how many floors up (except when carrying baggage, of course).
- Take along a protein balanced bar and an apple to help resist fast food
- Do not eat the sweet rolls at the free continental breakfast - eat the bowl of cereal instead with low fat milk or a yogurt.
- Take ear plugs in order to rest or take a nap
- Bring a tape or CD player to zone out to your favorite music
- Always order after you ask questions about content and get the salad dressing on the side
- Drink lots of water wherever you are.

Deep End

DRINK WATER

Working out in water and being careful about what you eat is critical to changing your chemistry for a healthy body. As it happens, drinking water in significant quantities should also be a regular part of your diet and exercise program. Here are some interesting and important things you should know about water.

Water has the following specific benefits:

- Suppresses appetite.

- Assists the body in metabolizing stored fat, because your liver is overloaded when your kidneys don't get enough water. Your liver metabolizes fat, and it can not do that at 100% efficiency if it is doing the job of the kidneys.

- Reduces fat deposits in the body.

- Relieves fluid retention problems. If you don't give your body water, it will hold water as a safeguard from losing it.

- Reduces sodium buildup in the body.

- Helps maintain proper muscle tone.

- Rids the body of waste and toxins.

- Relieves constipation.

Ideally, you should drink about 64 ounces or 2 quarts per day of clean water, preferably bottled or filtered. That is approximately 8 glasses of 8 ounces per glass. Yes, that sounds like so much water you may think you will drown. But the nice thing about water is that it is easy to drink. Colas or carbonated beverages actually take longer to drink because of the carbonation. Ever try to drink Coke fast? You could explode if you're not careful.

Now, the water experts advise that you should drink all this water and for every 25 pounds overweight you are, drink an additional 8 ounces per day. Another water drinking tip is to drink the water cold. Cold is absorbed into your body quicker and may burn more calories as the result.

Chapter 6: Aqua Healing

For many people water is about healing. Most of the people who come to my classes have been people who have come to the water out of necessity. They have concluded that there is simply no other practical alternative. In most cases they have tried just about everything conventional medicine has to offer including various drugs and chiropractic therapy. Some have even tried some not so conventional methods such as acupuncture or hypnosis. It is as though the idea of water is not something to be taken seriously and is only sought as an absolute last resort. Europeans accept water as a form of legitimate treatment for a variety of ailments, but Americans traditionally have not been so inclined.

Perhaps as a culture Americans have come to rely largely on the advances of science and medicine. Somehow to simply go in water is insufficient. Water exercise is just not sophisticated enough, particularly at this age in this high tech world. How could it possibly work? As a result water is often dismissed as an option.

Nonetheless, despite the ongoing skepticism about the effectiveness of water as a means to better health and to heal, many people each day are coming to the realization that water is very important to them. Roberta tells how water helped change her life of pain and discouragement, although she stubbornly resisted water exercise for months before giving it a try.

"I worked at a factory job that I thought was a good job for eight years. The last year I was there I was on light duty from a work-related injury. The injuries were to my neck, shoulders and upper back. When a doctor examined me, I had severe muscle spasms, trigger points, inflammation and my spine and ribs were out of alignment. I was put on anti-inflammatory drugs, muscle relaxants, pain medication and sent to a physical therapist. The drugs dulled the pain and the physical therapy gave me some relief. However, several hours after I left the office everything returned to the same condition as before treatment. Sometimes the effect of the treatment would last for several days. But the pain always returned.

"Weeks went by with me doing gentle stretches and exercises. I did find that some days I had less pain and muscle weakness. But little energy and little sleep had become typical. I continued to believe there would be light at the end this dark tunnel. I was wrong. I received notice that my workers compensation insurance decided I no longer had a valid claim and they would no longer pay for any treatment. I wanted to get an attorney to fight my battle, but I did not have the thousands of dollars to pay my bills. I was at my wit's end.

"The next six months became a nightmare of being harassed by my employer, trying to pressure me into quitting and I felt the walls coming in. What would I do without a job? How

117

could I help support the family if I could not support myself? How can I pay my bills? I became more and more depressed. All the while the pain only worsened because I could no longer afford any treatment. Being depressed certainly did not help.

"Just before I left my job, a friend suggested I try a certain chiropractor. I decided I had nothing to lose and scraped together the money I could to go see this chiropractor. At this point I hoped the chiropractor could not only provide some temporary relief, but also teach me about how my body worked and how to take better care of myself. The chiropractic adjustments gave temporary relief, but the exercises I learned only aggravated my injuries. I had periods of time when I felt better, then for no apparent reason, I would be back in the emergency room for pain medication.

"This cycle went on for several months. I did continue to see my primary care physician until all options with him failed. He had little to add except to try a deepwater exercise class at a local community pool. My reaction to this was: 'Why would this be any different?' His recommendation seemed pointless since I was convinced that I would really struggle in the water. And because I did not think I was comfortable in water, this would be the last thing I would do to get better!

"Next I tried tai chi floor exercises. I learned more about balance in my body and my life, just as my chiropractor had suggested I would. The philosophy of yin and yang made sense to me. But physically I was unable to maintain the exercises on a day to day basis. My frustration grew and at times my determination to get well left me in despair as the pain and depression returned. My doctor's frustration with me also grew and he invalidated my pain and invalidated me, suggesting that my pain was all in my head! After I expressed my despondency and hopelessness, he told me help was in more exercise not more pills. I said I want a reason why I hurt like this. What is my diagnosis? I said exercises make me hurt more each time I try to do more. With all the technology available and at his disposal why would he not try to find out what was wrong with me?

"I left the doctor without an answer. I looked deep into myself. This ordeal had left me with so much self-doubt. I tried to deny my pain or to acknowledge it. I reasoned that others had it much worse than me and look at their courage. I felt ashamed when I saw people wheelchair bound or with braces or walkers going on about their lives. How do they keep going? I have so little energy and so much pain. I am exhausted.

"I forced myself to continue some of the exercises and I tried a new job. If I could totally get into a new job, maybe I could keep my pain down. I turned a hobby into a job. I became a gardener for my church's summer camp. This I could do at my own pace. Then a chance encounter changed my life. I was working by the pool one morning and noticed the water aerobics class coming in. Many of the women were my age, others were a lot older, but all of them put on what looked like a rubber belt of some sort before they got in.

"'Were they all non-swimmers like me?' I wondered. This belt kept them afloat and they did not struggle to stay up. There was laughter and yet it looked like hard work. It appeared to be a solution to my exercise problems, but I dragged my feet for three more months before I investigated any further. By the time I collected my courage, the camp pool had closed. I had to find another pool. I was glad that finding another pool was not hard even in my medium size town. The three year-round pools all had water fitness classes. I returned to the one that had the friendly front-desk staff. I was introduced to the instructor and shown around the facility. Right away the people in the class shared with me and made me feel welcome and not so scared.

"There was a man partially paralyzed from a skiing accident, a woman who had fallen from a ladder and had crushed discs, several pre and post natal women, post surgeries, degenerative disc disease, fibromyalgia, and another woman who had a work related injury. Each looked confident and happy while in the water, and the ones who talked to me urged me to return. The instructor was supportive and upbeat while giving constant instruction. This was the most encouraged I had been since my injury. 'I could do this too!' I thought. 'I could belong to a group that was committed to doing something to have control in their life.'

There is nothing the body suffers which the soul may not profit by
– George Meredith

"Things were going to turn around. I was able to pace myself with my new job and have my own schedule and still get the work done. I changed doctors. I finally found a doctor to review my records and to arrange for me to have some diagnostic procedures. I took the plunge, both literally and figuratively. I knew I would finally get some answers. The next day I was in the pool with the group. After the first day I was so encouraged I decided to sign up for the class to help me commit.

"Three weeks after doing water fitness classes I felt a small sense of control returning. I was diagnosed (finally) with degenerative arthritis of the spine. Even though it was dreadful, I was actually relieved to find out this was not in my mind and not my fault. I would receive proper treatment and I was supported totally by my new doctor to continue water fitness classes. Within five weeks, I was no longer in need of the pain medications I lived with for several years. I felt stronger and was able to do more in my gardening job. I also slept through the night! I had more energy and my depression subsided.

"I am so glad I did not give up. I intend to make water exercise a permanent part of my weekly schedule for life. I am able to add walking and other recreational activities with my family now. This exercise program truly gave me my life back when I thought it was gone. I am able to enjoy life, family and work with its small pleasures again. I owe it to deep water and the instructor and to me for hanging in there."

Roberta's story is encouraging and people like her are one of the reasons I became addicted to water and impressed by what it can do for others. It is just heartbreaking to me when I hear of so many people who right now are suffering a variety of ailments and diseases that can be treated by using water. It is my personal mission to make as many people as possible aware of the wonderful benefits of water fitness. Conventional medicine serves its purpose. But there is much you can do for your health to prevent and treat without having to rely exclusively on your doctor and on drugs. Roberta is a good example of this. She is one of many people I have had the joy and privilege of working with in the water. To see people like Roberta undergo the miraculous changes brought on by working out in water is a thrill I would not give up for anything.

HISTORY OF HEALING

Water has been used for therapeutic purposes for thousands of years. Healing pools, baths, spas, and springs have been important to the therapeutic use of water. Water historian Jonathan Paul DeVierville notes that, "taking to water, soaking in baths and pools and resting at places called spas have played an important social and spiritual role in the river valley civilizations of Mesopotamia, Egypt, India, and China. Ritual bathing pools were widely used for individual, religious, and social renewal and healing. Healing water rituals also appeared in ancient Greek, Hebrew, Roman, Christian, and Islamic cultures. Ancient civilizations used the water for cleaning the earthly human body of disease and cleansing the spiritual body of sin. These cultures taught that clean bodies and pure souls facilitated seasonal as well as eternal renewal, which in turn ensured cultural regeneration."

Public baths and swimming pools were an important part of the culture of Rome. By the mid-4th century, there were about 1,000 public baths and swimming pools throughout the Roman Empire. One of the largest and most grand facilities was the Baths of Caracalla which could accommodate about 1,600 people and included a number of baths, swimming pools, exercise rooms, and lecture halls.

Swiss cultural historian Sigfried Gideon observed that "the manner in which a civilization integrates bathing within its life as well as the type of bathing it prefers, yields searching insight into the inner nature of that period… [in particular] the culture's attitude towards human relaxation. It is a measure of how far individual well being is regarded as an indispensable part of their community life."

Of course, there is much mysticism and folklore about certain water sources. Greek and Roman medical practitioners encouraged bathing in various mineral springs to cure a variety of ailments. Physicians of the Renaissance often prescribed specific spas or springs to treat specific ailments of the skin, skeleton, and organs. In Lourdes, France, the waters have for years been considered a source of miraculous cures of such things as arthritis, cancer, tumors, and the like.

Jonathan DeVierville points out that while claims for healing in some waters may be exaggerated or just plain fraudulent, there is legitimacy in the effectiveness of many water sources in which people soak. DeVierville asserts that there are a number of physical properties found in some natural water spas that can have very distinct health benefits. For example, sulfur, which is a natural bactericide, is found in some water sources and has shown various benefits on skin. In fact, many acne products are effective because of sulfur and the Army used sulfur to treat wounds right up to the 1940s.

Hot springs also stimulate circulation and your metabolism, which can treat rheumatoid arthritis. Many springs have carbon dioxide bubbles that also stimulate circulation (of course, the same effect can be achieved in a home spa with a bubble jet). Even springs that have a faint emission of radioactive radon can relieve arthritis. You don't have to seek out hot springs, though: a pool at a temperature of about 84 to 86 is effective for relieving arthritis.

In America mineral springs, spas, and just water as a therapeutic measure was only temporarily embraced in the past. As America expanded from the East to the West, pioneers learned about healing waters from Native American Indians. The industrious immigrants built spas around these waters. Then, as science, medicine, and technology began to bloom, particularly at the dawn of the 20th century, Americans began to lose interest in water as a source of healing. Most people perceived swimming pools, spas, and the like, as largely a luxury of the rich. Otherwise, water was for able-bodied people, and to a lesser extent, a small number of people afflicted with ailments such as arthritis. For at least most of the first half of the 20th century, the general American population did not associate being in water solely for fitness and health maintenance.

In Europe, however, water has always been a big deal. And these days going to a spa is a rather involved experience. You go to a rural setting for two or three weeks, take a series of special health promoting baths, eat a balanced diet, and engage in regular exercise to get your juices flowing. Europeans must be doing something right given that they generally are not as obese as Americans and are not nearly as prone to hypertension and heart problems.

Modern day American medicine does not automatically recommend water (hydro) therapy to treat various ailments. To prescribe hydrotherapy over the more conventional practice of drugs and surgery as a first step is unusual. Europeans make water an integral part of healing and health maintenance. With all the advantages we have in America, we have much to learn. Begin to think of water as a resource.

The Watering of America

I believe Americans are coming around to water. For one thing Americans are drinking more of it. John Spannuth, CEO of United States Water Fitness Association, notes that "water exercise is making a name for itself in all fitness circles for young and older, fit and unfit." Its versatility has researchers scrambling to study its effectiveness not only from testimonials but also from factual research. Water exercise provides benefits no matter what skill level. This is not a trend but an established form of exercise for the injured, sedentary, overweight, elderly and pregnant populations and now for the baby boomers. It is a

124

given that sooner or later we will experience an injury and need to have a way to heal ourselves. We are turning towards putting ourselves in water.

Americans are also drinking more water. Millions have become very particular and are starting to change the nature and quality of the water we drink. We are now doing everything from drinking expensive imported bottled water to buying special filtration systems to ensure that the water from the faucet is clean. Fortunately, there are some people in government who recognize the importance of water fitness as it relates to better health. To encourage Americans to go into water for better health and to accommodate those with existing ailments, the American Disabilities Act was enacted to finance public pools and ensure that new and existing public pools are accessible to anyone. Public pools are now designed to enable anyone to enjoy them, including those who are physically challenged or wheel chair bound.

Many new water fitness programs are being implemented throughout the country these days in public and private pools. Programs are springing up in community pools, at high schools, universities, country clubs, health spas and centers, and elsewhere. The YMCA in nearly every major and mid-sized city has been greatly instrumental in providing water fitness programs. For years the YMCA, in conjunction with the Arthritis Foundation, has provided water fitness programs for arthritis sufferers. Mary Essert, a YMCA water instructor and author of the *YMCA Manual for Special Populations*, stresses that the YMCA invites people to participate in their water fitness programs no matter what their fitness level. Essert took to water to treat her own chronic fibromyalgia and her breast cancer recovery. She says that they have a wide variety of people who join the YMCA

125

water fitness programs, from highly trained professionals to recent stroke or cancer victims. Nonetheless, YMCA water fitness programs are sometimes fragmented and there appears to be poor coordination of programs. But I still recommend the YMCA, especially in a city or town in which there may be no other option.

Despite the growing awareness of water fitness, a colleague and friend of mine, Dr. Bruce Becker, in his book, *Biophysiological Aspects of Hydrotherapy*, has pointed out that there is still much work to be done to educate people, especially Americans to the benefits of water. He writes: "aquatics is vastly underused. We have been lured by the appeal of high technology and advanced pharmacology often at the cost of greater medical expense and side effects."

WATER THERAPY

Water therapy may conjure thoughts of people recovering from surgery or an injury and being placed by medical technicians in some water tank or bath in a clinical hospital environment. But that is not necessarily true in most cases. Yes, there are specific forms of water therapy that you may want to do to treat a bad back, or an injured foot or arm, and I'll cover those things in this book. But water therapy can also mean a very pleasant way of treating yourself to a unique mind, body, and soul experience such as an herbal bath or a whirl pool or Jacuzzi. Water therapy can mean simply doing something special for you.

Pool Side

GETTING IN TUNE WITH YOUR BODY

Listen to your body as your fitness level develops. Women, it seems, tend to be more in tune with their bodies than men. There may be a variety of reasons for this. We have more to concern ourselves with, especially with respect to our monthly menstrual cycle. We are also concerned with our looks in a way that men are not. We worry about our hair, our clothes, and so on. Men don't. We seek hourglass figures. Men don't usually think as much about the way they look, what they wear, or whether or not they are in shape.

So, since women are more in tune with themselves than men, we seem more apt to identify things that are not quite right with us. But beware, we may have some chronic ailment or physical problem to which we can become indifferent. In other words, we can ignore some nagging ache or pain. I know of a number of women who just decided to ignore a pain in their chest, and ended up with a stroke. And I have known of other women who have ignored an ache in a breast and later discovered a tumor.

My aim here is not to alarm or frighten, but to draw your attention to your body and not to ignore anything your body is trying to tell you. I want you to acknowledge how important it is to be in tune with your body. I also want you to learn when an ache or pain is something you should be concerned about or something you know is the result of your workout.

Fortunately water fitness does not have the pounding impact that running, walking, or other land-based aerobics inflict. Instead, during your water workout the forgiving, buoyant effects of water always surround you. You will, however, feel an ache in your muscles, particularly in your arms, legs and to a lesser extent your back.

This is a good ache. If you follow my advice on the beginning water fitness exercise I outline, this will not be anything you cannot endure. The power of water is the overall strengthening gains it provides.

Muscle Builder

The fact is, as we exercise muscles we have not exercised for a long time, or perhaps exercise muscles for the first time, you actually create micro-tears to your muscle. Your muscles respond by producing lactic acid (which creates that aching feeling) and draw on special proteins that your body uses to build up your muscles. This is how your body attempts to repair the "damage" your workout has done and forces your body to condition itself as you continue to exercise. Your body builds muscle. In short, exercise increases muscle, tones your muscle, changes the chemistry of your muscle, and increases the metabolism of your muscle. As a result you burn calories at all times, even when you are not exercising. Every part of your body benefits.

But resting between intense workouts is critical to enable your body to recover. Generally, you do not have to be inactive after a hard workout, but you should have a little easier day following a hard workout day. You may also consider alternating one muscle group versus another muscle group every other day. For example, work your leg muscles hard one day, then give your upper body a good workout the next, and then go back to a lower body workout the third day, and so on.

Should you sense that you are overexerting yourself in a given muscle, put more emphasis on another muscle group for at least two to three days. This way you maintain your cardiovascular level and give the aggravated muscle a chance to recover. If you feel pain or discomfort after you continue with the overexerted muscle, evaluate your technique, posture, or whatever to determine what you may be doing wrong. If the problem persists, you may want to visit your doctor.

The key point here is to understand that relaxation is just as important to working out as the work out. It is another instance when balance enters the picture. Just as a balanced diet, we must balance our workout with hard days and easy days. Some of us are stubborn, and once we get going on a certain regimen, we don't want to stop. By allowing yourself to focus on all aspects of you, your mind, body, and spirit, you will recognize the value of listening to what your body is telling you. When you overexert, your body is saying: "Hey, slow down, relax!" And you better pay attention, or you may succumb to such pain or discomfort your body forces you to slow down.

Heart & Lungs

Other important muscles you exercise during your water workout are your heart muscles and lung muscles. You will not feel any ache or pain related to the toning of these muscles. Instead, you will notice, after several weeks, that your endurance level is greater. This is a very encouraging part of your regular workout. Your body is telling you that you are getting stronger and you can work out longer and at greater intensity, which leads to an even stronger, healthier, and leaner you!

Injury & Illness

Sooner or later an injury or an illness may challenge you. Your body responds by forcing you to slow down. You may be stubborn like I am, but you should not fight your body when it is telling you to take it easy. To deal with an injury or illness your body must use a certain amount of protein to take care of the problem. Any stress on the body, including sustained exercise, causes the healing and tissue repair process to slow down. You will find it harder to exercise at a higher level for which you have been conditioned.

When you have an injury or an illness it is advisable that you take it easy with your workout. This also applies to pregnant women. Rather than work out at 80% of your target heart rate, which we discussed in an earlier chapter, cut back your workout to perhaps 65% of your target heart rate. This ensures that your body not only helps you recover from an illness or injury, or possibly helps in baby development during pregnancy, but enables you to maintain your regular workout. And actually, by cutting back, you give your body a better chance to make you even stronger over time. Our bodies truly are remarkable.

If you experience pain while working out, the best thing to do is just stop. More than likely your body is trying to warn you of overexertion. Listen to your body. Here are some things to watch for:

- Nausea
- Extreme weakness
- A red face
- Breathlessness
- Excessive fatigue (very tired 3 hours after the workout)
- Chest pain or discomfort
- Lightheadedness or dizziness
- Focused musculo-skeletal discomfort
- Ataxic (unsteady) gait
- Confusion

If you experience any of these signs you should, walk slowly in place and inform your instructor or call your physician.

Herbal Baths

There are a variety of baths you can take that yield some nice benefits you probably would never have guessed. I am definitely a bath advocate and want to share several baths that have almost magical effects to soothe, to sedate, or even to stimulate. In her excellent and comprehensive book, *The Complete Book of Water Therapy*, Dian Dincin Buchman provides many tried and true remedies. Here are a few of my favorites:

Oatmeal bath

Therapeutic uses: to soften skin, overcome itchiness or hives, relieve sunburn, chafing, windburn, dishpan hands or diaper rash.

- Blend raw oatmeal into tiny particles. Add up to one cup oatmeal to tepid or warm bath water. You can purchase this prepared as Aveeno in the drugstore.

Salt bath

Therapeutic uses: to relax, release tension after too much sitting, for sluggish skin, and relief of menopausal symptoms.

- Use coarse sea salt to any bath to produce buoyancy and the feeling of relaxation. As little as a cup or two can be very calming for the body, totally relaxing and almost hypnotic. As little as 5 pounds of common coarse salt will approximate natural sea water which is between 1% - 7% salt.

This bath is good as a mild tonic on the body in the same way that bathing in the sea creates a feeling of mild euphoria. After a day of long meetings I find I can overcome that sluggish feeling of doing nothing. It is also one of my many weapons to help abort an oncoming cold. Salt holds heat very well. End the bath with a cooler shower.

Salt Glows

Women should do this with the changing of the seasons. Therapeutic uses include: eliminate dead skin, restore circulation, overcome sluggishness, and abort an oncoming cold.

- Make a paste with ground sea-salt in the palm of your hand. Then massage over unbroken skin, starting with your feet and legs, working up toward your heart. The friction of the salt on the skin acts as a body stimulant, increases the circulation in anemic conditions, helps to overcome mild depressions, increases the tone of the body before or after an infection, and can help to overcome the body trauma caused by drinking too much alcohol. This bath could be used in combination with the salt immersion bath.

Sage Bath

To stimulate your sweat glands for cleansing and detoxification purposes, try a sage bath. Buying these items in bulk at summer outdoor markets or health food stores reduces the expense. Grow your own sage and dry it for later use.

- As you are drawing your bath bundle up a handful of sage and let the water flow over it as the tub fills. Enjoy the warmth and sent of the outdoors while you cleanse your body. (To stimulate and increase your blood circulation, try a rosemary bath. Follow the same procedure as the sage bath.)

Apple Cider Bath

Apple cider vinegar is a reliable, inexpensive bath aid. It is easy to purchase in quantity at the grocery store. Keep it in decorative flasks by the tub. Therapeutic uses: combats fatigue, restore the natural acid covering of your body, detoxify, relieve itchiness of poison ivy or sun burn.

• Add about one cup to your bath. (Two cups to overcome itchiness.) To overcome fatigue I pour some in my hand and splash it over my shoulder, arms, back, and chest. Then I slide into the hot bath and soak. After a soak, I slowly let out the warm water and replace it with cold water that I splash over my feet.

Partial Sit Bath

Sit on a towel or rubber pillow in the tub. Therapeutic use: to help clear up respiratory congestion. Wear a T-shirt if you chill easily. Use tepid water, and get out of the bath as soon as breathing difficulties are somewhat eased.

Pine Bath

You do not need to chop down a tree, just use a readily obtainable liquid extract or tablet products from the Black Forest of Germany. These can be found in herbal or health food stores. Therapeutic uses: to open pores, get rid of rashes, and to stimulate the skin, eliminate blackheads, recovery after vigorous exercise, relieves breathing problems in asthma, bronchitis, helps overcome fatigue, induces relaxation, especially if you are unusually nervous.

- If the bath is intended to relieve fatigue after exercise, or to relax, fill the bathtub with water slightly lower than body temperature, 95-98 degrees. Pour in one capful of the pine extract. Immerse your entire body. Remain in the bath for 15-30 minutes.

- If you want to produce sweating, start the bathe at the above temperature, add the pine (follow the directions on the box of tablets), and increase the hot water to 102 degrees. Remain in the tub for 10 minutes. The aroma will make the bath feel luxurious, and pine will relieve muscle fatigue and aid in perspiration. Pine tends to induce perspiration.

Sulfur Bath

Natural sulfur waters have helped people to overcome a wide variety of skin ailments, and to heal the body internally as well as externally. Therapeutic uses: to treat skin problems, particularly to soothe skin, mild antiseptic, relieve pain in arthritis, treat acne.

- Fill the bathtub with tepid water (temperature is 95 - 102 degrees) and add from 1/2 to 1 1/2 cups of fine suspended particles of sulfur or sulfur-bath preparation. Call your drug store for this product or health food stores. (Although you can also try a borax or baking soda bath to make a similar bath.) Sit in the bath for 10-20 minutes. The sulfur is reduced chemically and is absorbed by the skin to produce its great healing, cleansing, and antiseptic effect.

Ascorbic Acid (Vitamin C) Bath

Hemorrhoids seem to be a common problem for the business traveler, office worker, as well athletes and dancers. The addition of ascorbic acid (which you can obtain in powder form from your health food store) bath greatly speeds up the healing process. Therapeutic uses: to treat some skin and sinus allergies, hemorrhoids, and skin infections.

- Pour 3 tablespoons in a warm bath during a sudden allergy attack.

- For relief of hemorrhoids, use a sit bath (shallow bath). Add 1 cup to 5 quarts of cool water. Sit in the bath for 1-15 minutes depending on your tolerance.

Hot/Cold Showers

You are probably thinking, "What? Cold showers? Are you nuts?!" But the fact is a cold shower is very good for reducing high temperatures to enable you to overcome fatigue.

How do you take a cold shower and survive? Start by running the water at a warmer temperature, and then make the water colder and colder to touch. Remember, when testing water temperature, using your hand is not the most accurate method. Instead, raise your leg into the stream of water to expose more surface area of your skin. When it feels cold to your leg, it is probably a little colder to your back or your belly. At this point, make the water a little warmer and then take the plunge and try to last for a count of ten, or about 10 seconds. With some practice, you can condition yourself to tolerate very cold water.

As an alternative to the quick cold shower, you can try the alternating hot and cold shower. This is a form of hydrotherapy effective for treating rheumatism, and certainly helps to reduce muscle inflammation, and to decrease the stiffness in joints. I also find that this method helps invigorate your blood circulation and enables you to overcome fatigue or just overall lack of energy. To use the hot/cold method, run the water warm first, then turn it gradually hotter. Make it hot, but not so hot that you scald yourself. Make it hot to touch on your hand, and jump in for a count of ten, or 10 seconds. Then, immediately change the temperature to cold. For some plumbing situations, there may be a momentary delay as your water source catches up with what you are doing. Now, tolerate the cold water for about a count of ten. Then try alternating between hot and cold several times.

Fun with Mr. Shower

You can get a hand held shower sprayer, such as my favorite Mr. Shower, which someone gave me for Christmas some years ago. Mr. Shower gives you more control over the shower stream of water. I enjoy taking the Mr. Shower and directing the shower stream at the soles of my feet for a powerful blast that immediately increases the flow of blood circulation at my feet. Using Mr. Shower you can practice reflexology by diverting blood from one part of the body to another part of the body, and thereby relieving congestion from the first part. The diversion of blood in this way is called a reflex connection. With the many reflex points on the soles of the feet, I think this application of water can be a very powerful form of treatment for some people.

You may also consider purchasing a hot foot bath from any drug store and use it to warm up from a chilly, rainy day or day of being on your feet. The benefits from the relaxation, warmth, and stimulation of the reflexology points are noticeable if given the chance.

Deep End

Miracles can happen, especially in water. Here are some reasons why.

EXPECTANT MOTHERS EXPECT MIRACLES IN WATER

Water is a great environment for pregnant women. The University of North Carolina at Chapel Hill conducted a study that demonstrates that working out in water three times a week reduces edema associated with pregnancy. Moreover, it was found that pregnant women who engage in a regular water workout could avoid pronounced varicose veins, especially in the lower extremities. And since a water workout while wearing an Aquajogger or similar equipment demands that you strengthen your abdominal muscles, this actually improves post natal recovery for women who maintain their water workout their pre and post natal period.

SENIORS FIND FOUNTAIN OF YOUTH IN WATER

Water fitness has been like a miraculous fountain of youth for many seniors. Seniors who make water fitness a regular part of their life find that they feel and are stronger, much more energetic than their non-exercising peers, and have a much more healthy and positive outlook on life. Erica Ziegler, the aquatic director at the Marin Jewish Community Center (San Rafael, CA), notes that water is "the great equalizer,' and that a water fitness program is good for seniors at "any age, at any stage." She says something I always tell people: "Water is very forgiving." Water is ideal for seniors because they can achieve a significant intensity level for their workouts without the impact of a land-based workout, and they can do this in the very supportive environment of water.

All this activity for seniors results in fewer medical problems and tends to increase their longevity. The other significant advantage for seniors is the social interaction that regular water workouts foster. Working out in water is a great social scene, and the workout is often the highlight of the week for many seniors.

After her husband died and a yearlong grieving period, Ethel knew she needed to change many things in her life. Getting into a smaller, less expensive living situation and improve her health with an exercise program was her first and second priority. She had gained a lot of weight through this traumatic period of her life and needed help right away. Rather than spend money for instruction she began to swim at her new apartment, but her commitment was minimal at best and the weather in the Pacific Northwest gives lots of excuse power to not following through! As her health (knees, hip and hands) started to limit her activities, her doctor insisted that she get her great 70 year old body into a serious exercise program at least three days a week.

"The water fitness class I started at the pool has been one of the most enriching situations I have ever gotten involved with. For 12 years I have consistently gone to class with the same instructor and many of the same people. Some of the best friendships I have ever formed have come from this class. Several people I have learned to "deal with" have helped me grow in my tolerance and appreciation for differences.

"We have to know our limits and stay within those boundaries to be a survivor. The same is true with water exercise. I have learned a lot about my body and mind while feeding my soul in these classes. Water exercise has been the renewing source for my body and my attitude every time I have had a setback with health issues, finances, and losing love ones. I always returned to the warmth of the water and what it does for my old body as well as

138

the caring people to renew my spirit. I experience a wonderful sense of calm after an invigorating workout. I feel even at 83 the water fitness class challenges and encourages me to fight the aging process!"

Paul began his entry into water fitness in the spring of 1997 on the recommendation of a friend.

"A few months earlier, and shortly after my 74th birthday, I had developed symptoms of coronary artery arteriosclerosis which required an angioplasty procedure. This took place in November 1996. I credit the water exercise class for helping me improve cardiac function and also with helping me drop and keep off 15 pounds of excess weight. As of this date, I have no further symptoms of coronary artery insufficiency.

"Because I felt so good after that recovery, I decided to do a remodeling project of our home in the years of 1997-1998 and seriously limited my water activity which aggravated and increased my arthritis symptoms. The rapid decrease of mobility, energy and range of motion from lack of *real* exercise led to a total hip replacement. Eight weeks after the surgery, I started once again in the water fitness class. My hip muscle strength improved weekly. It was possible to actually move the leg more easily at the end of each class.

"Within two weeks of resuming the class, I was forgetting to pick up my cane at the pool and the lifeguard would come running after me to return it. At the 12-week post-op appointment, the hip was strong enough that the doctor no longer required me to use a cane for regular walking. He praised me for my commitment to my water fitness class. There are so few people in my generation who even consider exercise as a way to better health and fitness."

WOMEN HAVE A CHANGE OF HEART IN WATER

According to Dr. Martha Hill, national past president of the American Heart Association, heart attack is the number one killer of American women. In fact, it is estimated that one in two women will eventually die of heart attack or stroke. This is a terrible statistic and there really is no reason why women should die of heart attack, especially when working out in water can prevent most heart conditions. I have had many women come to the water after surviving a stroke. They are extremely fortunate, and all of them know it.

If for no other reason, I strongly urge all women to consider water as a miracle cure to heart problems. We now know that if you have a damaged heart, you can reverse the process by working out in water. You can also strengthen your heart and lower your cholesterol level to prevent from becoming a victim to a diseased heart. Prevention, as they say, really is the best cure.

My mother, Marjorie, has been going to water exercise since she was 50 and was able to retire. She is now 73 and continues to go several times a week. My mother had been a stroke victim, but she knows the recovery has been helped through aquatic therapy and her commitment to her own personal water fitness program.

My mom also credits her water exercise as a way to enhance her balance in the water. Balance is something of great concern to older people. We younger people take balance for granted. Now, even though mom's community pool does not provide an instructor there are many committed people who meet 3 times a week at the pool for exercise. I have been many times to give them new movements and corrections. Mom is a very good womentor, and has encouraged many people to start water fitness using flotation belts.

140

Even my mother-in-law, Jean, is a regular participant at this pool. She has that positive attitude others like to be around. Often people do not even know she has her own physical challenges because she is so often helping others. The people down in the deep end are known as the Turtle Club by the lifeguards. Apparently the flotation vests they wear look like turtle shells they wear on their backs. I like that analogy because of how long sea turtles live, and how beautiful they are in the water, and how wise they always look. Please know you can be like a sea turtle and start your own club - all it takes is a fellow turtle aspirant.

Chapter 7:
Broadening Your Aqua Experience

You do not have to be a swimmer to benefit from water fitness. In fact, you do not need any special water related skills to benefit from water fitness. All you need is the right attitude and the willingness to begin and maintain a regular water fitness program. In time you will become comfortable and confident with your regular water fitness program. From there, you can plunge into other water-related activities or possibly add a land-based exercise to your regular weekly workout.

Vicki's Story

Most of the people who come to water fitness classes are not athletes. They are average people usually coming to water for any number of physical problems. Some of them become athletes, but most of them are happy just to get to the class regularly and keep themselves fit, healthy, and pain free. Occasionally, however, I do have an elite or professional athlete seek my services and this is always an interesting challenge for me. In most cases they have either very specific physical problems, or they are trying to make improvements on some sport-specific movements. Vicki is another shero of mine. She is a beautiful, healthy, single mom who is blessed with the determination to be an elite athlete. She has been a NCAA track champion and Olympian. She may look like a model, but she is really a mermaid disguised as a track star.

Vicki's career has included two NCAA championships and participation in two Olympic competitions. In 1988 she ranked as the sixth woman runner in the world. In 1996 she won the US Championship 1500 meter race and went to the World Cross-Country championship to run in the 3000 meter.

Vicki has achieved all this and you can find her on any given day, working out in the water and encouraging others just like everyone else. She relates as a womentor to young women to cross train and older women to keep the faith and not stop working out.

Not many women can say they work out with an Olympian. That is what is so great about water fitness. Many different levels of ability can work out at the same time, in the same space, at their own pace! Vicki motivates women three times her age while running three times as hard. She is always there to tell them to continue even though the effort may not come easily. She continuously encourages everyone by saying: "Don't stop believing you can do it!"

Vicki has been a regular water runner since college. She has used the water as her cross training component as well as the therapy portion of her rehabilitation. It has maintained her strength, sanity and aerobic capacity for competition through several bad injuries.

Vicki is back on the mend and getting ready to return to racing. She is an inspiration to many young women and also to women who continue to compete at her level even after having babies and turning 30.

DIVERSIFY YOUR WORKOUT

There are a couple of ways you can enhance your water fitness program. By either diversifying your workout in water or cross- training—adding a land-based exercise to your workout program—you can maintain your interest and fitness level more effectively.

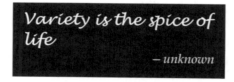

Variety is the spice of life

— unknown

Apart from just having fun in the water (which is a good thing, and I certainly encourage this!) you can engage in other water exercise to get a good aerobic or strengthening workout. Lap swimming is the oldest form of aerobic water workout exercise and involves swimming back and forth from one end of a pool to the other, employing various strokes (i.e., breaststroke, backstroke, etc.). Take lessons to improve your strokes. This will make swimming comfortable and efficient.

Water toning is another good water exercise, particularly if you want to stress aerobics combined with a strengthening workout to facilitate muscle toning. For the most effective water-toning workout you use such things as foam paddles, weights, or webbed gloves which you use in deep water or at the edge of the pool. These paddles and other special types of equipment are needed to create greater resistance as you move through the water. The resistance is what will make you stronger and the movement involved as you build strength makes the experience an aerobic workout.

Of course there are other ways you can work out in the pool and in a much larger body of water such as the ocean. Many people enjoy the movement and experience of surfing, scuba diving, or snorkeling. Just keep in mind that although these water activities do demand a certain amount of physical effort; it is much like the difference in effort between walking or a brisk run. One form of exercise is much more demanding than another, and like it or not, it is the demanding one that will be of greater benefit to you.

I suggest that you invest your time and effort into the more demanding activity, such as a vigorous water fitness workout, and engage in the other water activities for fun. As a comparison, this would be like running seven or eight miles four times a week (for a vigorous workout), and playing tennis for fun. At least you will know that playing the tennis or surfing or whatever will be much easier and more enjoyable because you are in better shape through your regular, much more strenuous weekly workouts.

Cross-Training

Diversity is a good thing. Nearly any experienced, open-minded workout instructor acknowledges the benefits of cross training between distinctly different types of exercise even if the instructor has her own personal preference. Cross-training is a good idea because the fact is that no matter how strenuous your workout may be for a given exercise, you are not going to exercise certain muscles that another *different* exercise can.

Besides, our bodies naturally love a challenge and react differently to various stimuli. We are actually designed for more

145

physical activity than our sedentary lifestyles demand. By engaging in a variety of physical workouts, we will have greater muscle symmetry and also feel that our body and spirit are improving as a whole.

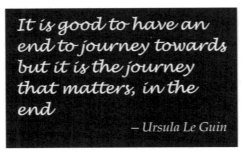

It is good to have an end to journey towards but it is the journey that matters, in the end

— Ursula Le Guin

A good argument for an elite land-based athlete to cross train with water is that it prevents potential injuries from overuse of the same muscles while maintaining strength and aerobic endurance. Another advantage to the land-based athlete is that water slows down motion, enabling the athlete to concentrate on sport specific movements. For example, runners are very strong in their legs, particularly in their quadriceps, and to a somewhat lesser extent in their calf muscles. But should the runner add bicycling as a regular part of her weekly workout, she will notice that her calves will become much stronger. Consequently, her stronger calf muscles will improve her overall performance as a runner.

So, here is a brief summary of reasons why I encourage water dancers to eventually cross-train, most likely with a land-based exercise:

- You strengthen certain muscles and ligaments not emphasized in your water workout, plus you enhance muscle symmetry
- You build endurance on land
- You build confidence that you can do anything
- You keep things interesting for yourself by adding variety
- You make new friends in your cross-training activity

Choosing the Best Cross-Training Exercise

As a water dancer, your water fitness program is a very good place to start towards developing a cross-training fitness program. By starting in the water, you can gain confidence at your own pace. Then you can consider what type of activity would interest you for cross training. Everyone likes different activities for different reasons. What may be good for your friend may not be good for you. You have to think about what you may like to try and then go out and try it!

Some people like to walk. Brisk walking is a very good aerobic workout and I encourage anyone to do it. Walking is really good for people who have never done any exercise before in their lives. Other people may try running because they simply want to challenge themselves or they don't have the patience for walking. Other people will prefer riding a bike because this seems more fun to them, while walking is boring to them, and running is just too hard on their limbs. I know people who enjoy rowing a boat, so they got themselves a rowing machine. Maybe you are an indoor sort of person, and you could not be bothered with all these other activities, so you get yourself a stair-climbing machine, or a cross-country skiing machine, or a stationary bicycle.

Note that the activities I just mentioned are among the best and most popular types of continuous aerobic exercise. And this is an important thing to bear in mind when selecting your activity. You should try to select an activity that is truly steady and aerobic to achieve the greatest benefit in your cross-training program. Here are some of the most efficient types of exercises grouped according to aerobic efficiency:

Most efficiency	Medium efficiency	Lowest efficiency
Jumping rope/jacks	Walking	Swimming
Running	Bicycling	Stationary bicycling
Chair/Stair stepping		Ice/In-line skating
Rowing		
Cross-country skiing		

The activities that many people enjoy, but are the least efficient aerobically, and are mostly non-aerobic, include many of the most popular stop-and-go or low intensity sports including tennis, football, handball, weight lifting, sprinting, square dancing, yoga, horseback riding, weight training, volleyball, and golf.

Additional Strength Training

As you engage in a regular water workout, you will get stronger. Your arms, your legs, your back, your shoulders, your neck, and so on will get stronger. However, you can augment your strength training in several ways to improve your performance in or out of water.

As I mentioned earlier, the most effective means to strengthening in water is to learn to catch the water with your palm or pointed toe. Equipment is secondary. The resistance is what makes you stronger, but if done properly, you can also strengthen through a land-based weight-training program. I recommend a book by Thomas Farley *Basic Weight Training For Men & Women, 2nd Edition* (Mayfield Publishers, 1994), which provides some good, basic weight training exercises. I also encourage you to take a weight training class or to hire a personal trainer to teach you safe and effective training to get you started.

For now, I will offer a simple strengthening exercise for your triceps. I am not suggesting that you develop huge, masculine muscles, but rather you can achieve lean, contoured and toned muscles. Triceps should do 65% of the work with lifting.

First purchase inexpensive bar bells, each at least weighing two pounds, working up to 5 pounds. Then follow these steps:

1. With weight in each hand, palms up, elbows bent. Stand with feet apart about the width of your shoulders, bending knees slightly.
2. With your back straight, curl the dumbbells back (extend backwards). Support may be aided by leaning on opposite leg. Do one arm at a time.
3. Curl dumbbells half way to your chest and lower.
4. Curl dumbbells all the way to your chest and then lower. This represents one rep. Lower your dumbbells slowly, contracting your arm muscles tightly to ensure good intensity.
5. Rest for a minute and repeat another rep as described. Repeat reps until you can't do it anymore for best results.

Eventually, as you get stronger, you may want to purchase heavier weights and increase repetitions. In addition to this simple triceps routine, there are many other weight-training exercises you can perform to strengthen and tone all major muscles.

Pool Side

WHAT IS GOOD FOR ELITE ATHLETES
IS GOOD FOR YOU!!

Most people would be surprised if they knew how many professional and elite athletes have made water an important and routine part of their workout. Granted, in many cases, even these athletes started with their land-based training only to discover the benefits of water training because of an injury. However, in nearly every case, after the injury had healed, these athletes continued with their water exercise to continue reaping the benefits of a high resistance, low impact workout in water.

A Kansas City Royals professional baseball pitcher had severe tendonitis of his pitching elbow and an injured rotator cuff. He underwent water training by pitching in water up to his neck with and without a resistive cord. He eventually returned to the game strengthened and rejuvenated. Olympic ice skating champion, Nancy Kerrigan rehabilitated a knee and thigh injury in water and continued to practice figure skating jumps and maneuvers without risk of injury.

Over the years, many coaches and athletes have automatically included water workouts as part of their training. They know that nearly any sport-specific movement can be simulated in water. Mohammed Ali and Rocky Marciano both enhanced their boxing speed and agility by regularly working out in water. Members of the Dallas Cowboy football team work out in water to improve strength and agility skills. Three-time Olympic gold medallist track athlete, Jackie Joyner-Kersee made tethered water running part of her workout. Nine-time Olympic gold medallist pentathlon athlete, Carl Lewis works out in the water and even practiced balancing exercises in front of the flume of a forced-water jet.

> Whether you use a bat, a tennis racket, a golf club, or have some other sport-specific movements, you can improve and enhance your performance in water. Does this mean actually going into a pool with a bat, or a golf club, or whatever to practice? Yes, that is exactly what people do to take advantage of water to improve their performance for a specific sport.

Water Yoga & Water Tai Chi

I always want you to understand the importance of combining your workouts with relaxation. A good aerobic workout can give you energy and can also induce a certain calm over you. Meditation can certainly facilitate relaxation and I believe meditation can be an important part of your mind, body, and soul workout.

In addition to meditation, you can also add an occasional extracurricular activity for fun that can help you relax in water. The latest thing, which is actually something that has been around for centuries, is yoga and tai chi. The new twist is doing very similar land-based yoga and tai chi movements in water. Not all pools offer a class or regular program that include water yoga and tai chi, but you could take a land-based program through a local community college or the YMCA, and then transfer your knowledge to the water on your own. There are some books on the subject, too. But I always encourage you to take a class, to get good instruction, meet new people, and most importantly, relax and have fun.

MAKING THE MOST OF YOUR DIVERSE WORKOUTS

To benefit most from a workout program that includes varied water exercise combined with land-based workouts, it is im-

151

portant to keep things interesting, you are exercising different muscle groups, and you are trying to keep things fun and relaxed. Because if you don't avoid boredom, and you don't have fun, and you don't relax, you will not keep up your fitness program.

I suggest that your program include water fitness with varied activities stressing different muscles alternately each session, three or four times a week. Also, alternate your water fitness with a land-based exercise. Try to do the land-based aerobic exercises two or three times per week. Ideally, a couple days of these aerobic exercise days should include some land-based weight training.

Keep in mind, what I am suggesting here is an ideal, and something you work towards. I would not expect anyone to start with such a regimen in the first week, or even the first month. But it is an ideal that you can strive for in the future as you get stronger, gain confidence, and feel better about your progress.

Deep End

SENIORS: MIND, BODY & SOUL FITNESS IN WATER

For many seniors, frail, or unconditioned people just doing daily activities like climbing a flight of stairs, turning a doorknob, getting up from a chair, and maintaining balance while walking means experiencing a better quality of life. And as our population gets older, these are going to increasingly become concerns for many more people in the years ahead. Although many people will find it difficult to engage in the normal activities of life as they get older, water can change all that.

Water is an easy medium in which to perform most movements because of its buoyancy. By exercising in water, strength returns due to the resistance, and before long, the once weak person is able to resume normal activities on land.

Here are some simple water exercises you can do or teach others to do to improve their quality of life:

1. Walking can be improved in the water. Emphasize good posture and walk in different directions. Begin by walking several minutes forward, several minutes backward, and walking sideways, left for several minutes, and then right for several minutes.

2. To improve balance, particularly for walking, hold a kick board at the surface of the water with each arm. Walk in the pool as described above, using the kick board to maintain your balance as you walk.

3. Climbing stairs can be practiced in water by climbing actual stairs emerged in the water on the side of the pool, or by walking and doing squats holding onto the wall.

4. To enhance strength in fingers, forearms, and wrists, to make simple motor functions easier to open doors, turning knobs, opening packages, cooking, etc., begin by touching finger tip to thumb in a circle then stretch back. Repeat with each finger. Spider push ups right to left finger, tips stretching. Flex and extend wrists, 5 slow/15 fast, and grasp small objects under water. Flex and extend elbow, 5 slow/15 fast, and grasp small objects under water.

153

5. In neck deep water (or a squat position in shallow water), cross your arms in front of your chest, alternating the left arm over the right arm and then the right arm over the left. Also stretch out towards a "pot" to pick it up and bring it back to you.

6. Getting up from a chair can be practiced in water by standing in waist deep water with legs, shoulder-width apart, and slightly bent. Your forearms should be flat on the surface of the water, palms down. Now, as you rise by straightening your knees, push your palms down into the water. Once you have straightened yourself, slowly bend your knees, and as you do, bring your hands up, palms up, from under the water to the surface. Repeat. Do this for several minutes.

As we all age, being able to care for themselves does a great deal to improve their self-confidence and sense of independence. Getting stronger with water can literally change the attitude and outlook seniors have on life. There are few reasons why anyone should suffer the indignities and sense of helplessness because they cannot do things they used to do with ease. A regular water workout can change their lives by giving them strength and greater mobility and in effect giving them their lives back.

Chapter 8: Aqua Men

Men make up a small percentage of the people who come to my water fitness classes. I think men are under the impression that water fitness is not manly enough. They associate "real" working out with sweaty, grubby land-based activities where you literally "feel" some impact. They can relate to sports like basketball, football, and hockey because they are sports where brawn, strength, grit and "masculine" characteristics are displayed. That's why dancing is generally shunned by men. Dancing is not manly enough. Dancing is for wimps. There is no overt sweatiness or grime or display of masculinity in dancing. Likewise, I think men have shunned water fitness for the same reasons.

MOST COMMON OBJECTIONS FROM MEN

I have heard men express concern that they would not get as good a workout in water as they would on land. How can you compare running, jumping, throwing balls, and the like to splashing around in water?

The theory that you don't get as a good a workout in water versus traditional land-based activities is simply not true. The resistance of water alone is enough reason for any man to realize that water is an excellent medium for getting a good workout. The fact is, in many ways, as I have shown elsewhere in this book, working out in water demands much more of our bodies than on land. But perhaps an objection to water is because men think they don't sweat? In a sense, you really *do* sweat in water; you just don't feel it the same way.

Embarrassment

Some men object to water fitness because they are embarrassed to wear swimming trunks and expose the rest of their body for the world to inspect. The fact that they are out of shape and possibly obese may be especially embarrassing to them. Many might argue that at least at a gym or while engaged in some sport, you could conceal yourself for the most part with T-shirts or other sporting apparels.

This may be a legitimate concern. Believe me, though, most people are thinking more about what *they* look like in their swimsuit than *you* do. Besides, there is no reason why a man can not wear a T-shirt or terry robe to and away from the water. And, of course, once you are in the water no one can see what you look like anyway. Eventually, as you get in shape, you won't have anything to be embarrassed about and can proudly exhibit yourself in the sleekest Speedo brief money can buy.

Then there is the embarrassment of possibly being seen splashing around in a pool with a bunch of women. After all, what is a man going to do if he's the only man in the pool? Won't he feel awkward and a little out of place? If you are a single man, this may not be such a bad situation. Single women make water fitness a regular part of their lifestyle and this shows a man that such women are concerned about getting in shape and being in shape. This is also what a woman will think about a man. Even if a man is not single, going with his wife or girlfriend is a good way to work out together in a very supportive environment. I always encourage wives to bring their husbands.

Generally, any man who goes regularly to a pool is welcome, encouraged and supported by the women at the pool. It is in the nature of 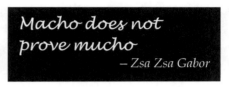 women to nurture and encourage. In this unique environment of water fitness for better health, people (both men and women) are particularly supportive. I think it has something to do with the "I've been there" mentality. Also, of the men that do come to the pool, I am seeing some well-conditioned athletic men who come to cross-train in water. This can be encouraging to a man when he sees other men taking water fitness seriously.

Macho does not prove mucho
— Zsa Zsa Gabor

Time

The apparent lack of time for a regular workout program of any kind may be one of the greatest objections among men *and* women. The biggest excuse I hear is that work interferes with the time they might have to exercise.

I believe if most men are honest with themselves, they will admit that work and career is the most important part of their lives. This even applies to men who insist that other things are more important such as their spouses, children, and so on. Unfortunately, I have known men who have virtually sacrificed their own physical, mental, and spiritual well being because of work. They rationalize with a "You have got to get the job done at any cost!" attitude.

There is nothing wrong with work. At times, even I may be accused of being a workaholic. What is misdirected is the priority placed on work over one's own health, physically, mentally, and spiritually. A man must ask himself what is really important?

Heart disease is still the biggest killer of men (and women) in the U.S. and in most industrialized countries. It is a known fact that heart disease is incurred to a large extent by poor diet, lack of exercise, and persistent anxiety or stress. In most cases, more than likely, the lack of exercise and anxiety part of the equation is directly related to work. If we are so willing to sacrifice ourselves for work, we have to ask ourselves what good is it if we drop dead in the process? Working can be an investment into you, as in building a career. Likewise, if investing in yourself through work is so important, doesn't it make sense for you to invest in your own health to enjoy the fruits of your labor?

I figure we all can find time to eat, brush our teeth, shave, bathe ourselves, sit in front of the tube for hours, and so on. We do this because we *make* time for these activities. I suggest you evaluate your life and decide if it is not time to make time for an investment into yourself. Even if all you can spare is as little as 30 minutes of working out per session, three times a week, I guarantee, it will make a huge difference in all aspects of your life. You may even realize that staying fit can actually help you perform better at work.

GOOD REASONS FOR MEN TO BECOME WATER DANCERS

Here are just a few of the reasons why men should reconsider water:

Strengthening and toning/lose weight
Increases endurance
Improves flexibility
Low impact/low injury
Helps reduce risk for prostate cancer
Reduces pain and swelling of arthritis
Improves sex drive
Induces calming and relaxation
Lowers risk for hypertension and heart disease
Improves sleep
Enhances mental capacity and alertness
Good social experience
Wonderful way to share time with spouse or girlfriend
Improves sport-specific movements, like golf or tennis swing
Not sick as often because of bolstered immune system
Helps you look younger
Good place to get in touch with your spiritual side
Balance and coordination
Longevity

If you choose to be open-minded, and consider the possibilities of water fitness as an alternative to land-based only exercise, you are more likely to appreciate the benefits. Like many women, most men become converts to water fitness out of necessity, and as a last resort. It's usually what ails them that practically force them to go to water to deal with their problems.

Other men come to water fitness via a coach or the advice of a trainer or fellow athlete. These are more likely trained athletes; water fitness becomes a regular part of their training to take advantage of the low impact, high aerobic, athletic career-extending benefits of water.

Then there are a smaller percentage of men who come to water fitness because of their partner, a spouse or a girlfriend. Like anything else when dealing with men, it is important not to nag a man (or anyone for that matter) to go to water. You would not want to say: "Hey, you old goat, you look like a wreck. You need to get your lazy butt to the water fitness class!"

> *In our civilization, men are afraid that they will not be men enough and women are afraid that they might be considered only women*
>
> — *Theodor Reik*

It is much more effective to serve as an example to a man. Seeing you make water fitness a part of your life and the effects of water fitness in your life can be very encouraging. At some point, you may invite him to tag along just to see the facilities. You are not looking for a commitment, just exposing him to the environment. While there you say something like: "Doesn't that look like fun?" To which he will probably retort: "No." And you might respond by telling him that if you did it together, it could be fun. And he might say: "Maybe."

Be patient with a man when it comes to water fitness and he may just come around. And when he does come around, encouragement is the most important thing you can do for him. Never be critical. Do the woman-man mentoring thing. Always seek to support and encourage. Like women, men need to feel that they are doing well, even if everyone else around them

160

seems stronger or more capable. The important thing is that he perceives you are proud of him and his effort to do something to be fit and healthy.

Doug's Inspirational Story

Doug is one of those kinds of guys who probably would never have considered water fitness unless he was injured. But like so many men like him, once in the water, they never want to quit.

"Six years ago, I suffered a herniated disc in a work related injury. I was pulling the green chain (sorting lumber) in a saw-mill when my accident occurred. I started a physical therapy class five years ago. But my treatment/therapy was over long before the pain and constant aggravation ended. Desperate to deal with the persistent pain, I considered water fitness. I found the back conditioning class that Juliana teaches at Sheldon Pool and I attend three times weekly. At this point, I have avoided back surgery. The water workouts have had a tremendous strengthening and healing effect on my back unlike anything else. I know I have lots of room for improvement, but I am able to keep the pain at a manageable level with regular water fitness.

"I feel being in the water to work out has allowed me to increase my flexibility and range of motion without the increase in pain that I often experienced with my physical therapy sessions. I also feel that I have learned pacing skills in the water fitness class that carry over to my day to day routine. Juliana is always nudging me to do a bit more, stay a bit longer and increase the repetitions on my stronger days. I have learned to change my bad habits of putting undue strain on my back muscles. And I have noticed an improvement in my posture and my ability to do my part time job as a sound engineer for church services and concerts of the church I attend.

"When I started this class, I couldn't even do the basic land exercises my doctor had recommended without a lot of pain. Even in the deep-water class I have experienced some discomfort during some of the exercises, but I know that this is only a warning sign and not a reason to stop water fitness. I learned how to modify and slow my movements while still maintaining the strength building component of the exercises. I have strengthened my back and have avoided further injury. I am cautious but am doing more than I have in years.

"My personal goal is to be able to lift 70+ pounds correctly in a work situation. I feel I can achieve this goal if I keep coming to the water fitness class consistently and continue to increase the resistance with increased speed and resistive equipment.

"One thing I can say with absolute conviction is that water fitness can help people with back injuries whether they are working on their own or as part of a return to work program. I am glad that I chose to be open-minded enough to give water fitness a chance. All you need to do is try it. You will be amazed how it can literally change your life."

Doug has been an encouragement to other men to consider water fitness as an excellent workout medium. And I believe that as more men come to the water, this will draw even more men like a magnet.

Pool Side

MEN IN WATER

Most men love a gadget (of course that is not to say women do not). I'm sure it has something to do with a man's innate visual orientation and his need to fix things. A gadget is usually the result of finding a way to fix a problem—to make something work. So ladies, get your guy an electronic, waterproof wristband heart monitor to help him keep track of his heart rate while working out. Heart monitors have an electronic display and several buttons to press—guy stuff. Some are pretty simple; others are remarkably sophisticated.

The advantage of a heart monitor is that it enables you to more accurately workout at a good fat burning, calorie burning aerobic rate. After all, if you are not working out at your most efficient aerobic rate, what's the point? Granted, not everyone can afford an electronic heart monitor and some people (including some men) don't want to fuss with a gadget. But for those people who can afford a heart monitor and enjoy fussing with gadgets, it's a good investment to make.

There are basically three types of heart monitors: Continuous read monitors, Zone monitors, and Downloadable monitors. A Continuous read monitor is the most basic as it simply displays your heart rate (price range: $69 to $100). Zone monitors are the most popular and they let you program your target zone into the monitor. As you workout a little beep or flashing icon displays on your monitor telling you where you are in the target zone. There are a variety of models with various features, so check them out (price range: $100 to $200).

Then there are the Downloadable monitors that are for the very technically oriented. You can not only program your target zone, count calories, or provide the percentage of your maximum heart rate, but you can download your data into your computer to manipulate (price range: $200 to $700).

Deep End

MEN: MIND, BODY & SOUL FITNESS IN WATER

I personally think that women are equally as competitive than men, but I know that men are often thought to be more competitive because of their testosterone level. So, I suppose I can appeal to the competitive side of men when I tell them that I know how they can improve in water nearly any form of competitive sport they enjoy.

Suppose you are a tennis player and you want to improve your game. Obviously you would not be playing tennis at all if you did not already know how to hold the racket, serve the ball, volley the ball over the net, and so on. But what can improve your game has a lot to do with attitude and confidence, not just mechanical ability. This is the mental and spiritual side of the game. This side of the game is just as critical to playing as knowing the mechanics of the game. In water, you can physically condition yourself for tennis and at the same time you can build on your mental and spiritual side in a way that you can't on land.

The advantage of water fitness in tennis and other sports is that you can achieve improved physical performance through water resistance strengthening exercise without strain or injury because you are in water. Flexibility and agility is also enhanced, plus certain specific hand, wrist, and arm movements can be improved in water. The lack of impact enables you to repeat the same sport-specific movements zillions of times without risk of injury.

Meanwhile, through ongoing meditation, concentration, visualization, and affirmation exercises you perform while working out, you enhance your mental and spiritual capacity of being focused and developing greater concentration. Focus and concentration will directly affect your reaction time on the court. And as you see yourself improve on the court, this will build confidence. Ultimately, you will be a better player.

Many men are golf fanatics, and much of golf, like tennis, is very mental and spiritual. Trying to remain calm and focused is critical to performing well in golf. Again, water fitness enables a golfer to improve his game in all these areas.

The fact is, there are professional athletes in nearly every sport who make water fitness a part of their training. Tennis players, golfers, boxers, gymnasts, football players, basketball players, soccer players, hockey players, baseball players, and so on take to the water to improve their games.

MAKE A DATE WITH YOUR MATE IN THE WATER

For those of you who have husbands or boyfriends that are already fairly athletic, it may not be difficult to get them to join you at the pool at least every once in a while. Working out in water with someone you love and care about can really be a fun and special time together. Going together occasionally can be a good thing to do on a date.

Donald Black, dating/relationship expert and author of *Smart Dating: A Guide to Starting & Keeping a Healthy Relationship* strongly advises that people who are already in an established relationship continue to date. That dating should not end once you are married or have decided to live together. Dating is a special time just for the two of you and helps maintain the bond that keeps you together. Instead of a movie, try going to a local hotel or a resort out of town, check in and go work out in the water! It's unique and different and fun.

What follows are a couple of exercises you can do with your partner to make the time together in the water a good, fun workout.

Kick Board Race

Everyone has seen a kick board. But in case you have not, a kick board is a small, floatable Styrofoam board (shaped a little a surfboard with one end chopped off), maybe a foot wide and a couple of feet long. Get a couple of these, one for each of you. Kick boards can be found in any pool supply place or the swimming department of Walmart or some similar establishment.

Then you and your honey get into the pool and do a little stretching. Once you have stretched and warmed up for about ten minutes or so, you are ready for the first event: the kick board race.

You start your kick board race at the shallow end, standing. Grab the kick board at one end, lengthwise in front of your body, and use whatever kick you need to race your partner to the other end of the pool and back. You race each other or time for speed or whatever. Do this a few times and you will definitely get your heart rate up.

Double Water Wheel

This is a little more complicated, but it can be fun making it work. I borrowed this from Jane Katz' water fitness book, *The New W.E.T. Workout*.

To get started, you should both float side by side in back layout position in opposite directions (head to toe, toe to head). Each

166

partner bends the right knee, with right instep against the inside of the left knee.

Each person holds partner by left ankle with his/her hand. Using the right hand for figure-eight sculling, and keeping it close to your hip, move "wheel" around in a circle in the direction of the best knee. Once you figure out how to get started, this can be a blast to goof around. And by the way, you do get your heart rate up in the process, which is good.

Water Massage

No, I'm not referring to the shower head application for a water massage, I'm talking about you and your partner taking turns massaging each other in the water. This could be a cool down you do just before you get out of the pool.

To do it right, begin by standing in shoulder deep water. Your partner should be positioned behind you. Then your partner massages you gently beneath the water surface using the heels of the palms. Be careful about grinding your palms into your partner's spine, this is not a comfortable feeling. Using the gentle pressure of a thumb along the muscles on either side of the spinal cord is also a nice technique. As your partner massages you, just relax, close your eyes, inhaling and exhaling slowly. The water/massage combination is a wonderful feeling.

Afterwards, when your both wrapped cozily in warm thirsty terry robes, and you have that calm relaxed yet invigorated feeling of having been in water, who knows what might happen back in your room.

Chapter 9: Aqua Inspiration

My purpose from the very beginning with this book has been to do more than simply provide a laundry list of exercises. There are plenty of good books on the market that provide water fitness instruction and technique (several of them are listed at the end this book for you to consult). Instead, my aim has been to provide direction, encouragement, and inspiration. I want to show you that fitness should not be limited to just exercising your body, but that you can "exercise" your whole life.

The fact is I have rarely met anyone who made exercise an important and integral part of their life and did not experience changes in other areas of their life directly or indirectly related to exercise. For example, when you exercise you start developing a concern over the food you eat and its nutritional content. Naturally, with all your physical effort, why would you throw it all away by continuing to eat junk? Certain habits like smoking begin to seem more ridiculous. You also discover that you have more energy to do things. So, you end up doing more. Your attitude becomes more positive and your overall frame of mind calm.

You may think how wonderful all this sounds. But I know that taking that first step toward making a lifelong commitment to exercise is the most difficult thing to do. I have learned over the years that the most effective way of getting people committed to regular exercise, especially a water fitness program, is to develop relationship. You will meet a pool full of people happily engaged in water fitness activities. You are bound to find at least one person you can relate to! Remember never swim alone. Take a buddy. Or find a buddy there. In this book, we have the next best thing; personal accounts of people who have made a commitment to water fitness. This chapter is devoted entirely to these personal accounts.

CAROL'S STORY

Carol is one of my best friends; I have known her most of my life. We have always kept in touch, but it had been years since we had seen each other. It was wonderful to see her again at our thirtieth high school reunion. We had a slumber party for several of us because we just couldn't get enough of each other. Carol and I, along with our friend Mary, had a lot of fun reminiscing. We even cried a lot together, reflecting on all the years and events that had gone by.

What is neat about Carol is that she is one of those few people who have known me ever since I was a child. This makes our relationship extra special. We both grew up in the same town and went to the same school from fourth grade right through high school graduation. We both married our high school sweethearts the same year, 1969. I was the lucky one as my relationship with my husband grew stronger over the years, while her relationship with her husband fell apart. She was sad about the whole situation, mad about the lost time, but very grateful for the two super girls she and her husband had together.

After her marriage, Carol became very open to trying some new things, and, although she was a Southern girl, she was even interested in learning more about the West Coast perspective on life. Generally, Carol was trying to determine what her future might hold and what alternatives were out there for making change in her life. She told me that it was finally going to be her life and not one for a husband or one for the kids. Now she had the opportunity to go her own way.

Carol has a lot going for her. She is well educated, is attractive with a slim figure, and has always been an upbeat person. She is also a nurturing and compassionate person. Despite these advantages, Carol knew it was going to be a long road back to being her old self. She had lost a lot of her self-confidence as most women do through a divorce.

As we talked, the thing that piqued her interest more than anything was water fitness. Perhaps I blew her away with my passion for water. I don t know. But she definitely got some positive vibes about water and just wanted to know everything. I happily obliged. Carol explained to me that she never really had a workout program before, but she wanted to change that, because there were other activities she wanted to do but wasn t strong enough. She was very interested in being strong and not having so many painful days with her knees and fibromylagia. These two conditions got in the way of most of her "fitness club ideas" of getting fit, enjoying outside recreation and meeting new people.

Before we had our heart to heart talk, Carol felt there were stumbling blocks in many aspects of her life. As far as getting her started on a regular water fitness program, it just so happened that I knew a great instructor in our home town, Pat Marandy. Pat is at the University of Alabama (my Alma mater). After our wonderful time together, I went home and Carol went right to Pat's water fitness class and registered. Carol tried it out and quickly became hooked.

The water fitness class was just what Carol needed. First she was encouraged that the non-impact workouts in water did not give her knees any pain. This made the exercise enjoyable in a way that she could not experience on land. Without pain associated with the exercise, she soon realized that water fitness not only gave her the strengthening workout she wanted, but also helped her unwind and to deal emotionally and mentally with the daily grind in her work of teaching young kids. Carol also found the water fitness class socially rewarding, particularly since the women who attend are such a diverse and interesting group. This has helped Carol a great deal in coming to terms with her feelings about the end of her marriage and looking forward to what the future holds. The womentoring in her water fitness class has helped Carol find the strength within and the courage to go on with confidence.

Carol and women like her have taught me much about their personal challenges. I have developed a special appreciation and respect for all women I know who rediscover themselves after a divorce or death of a spouse.

Carol loves the challenge of working out now. She also inspires and is inspired by her group who comes a long way after work to make a commitment to fitness. It is so exciting when you can be part of making a dramatic positive change in someone else's life, especially someone you love and care about.

MARY'S STORY

Mary can honestly say that water fitness has completely changed her life. Her story begins with her business and how it ruled her life. Mary has been a successful beautician for over 25 years. In fact, her business was so good that it left very little time for much of anything else, although she pushed herself to attend to her family, housework and playing with the dogs. But Mary was overextended trying to run a thriving business, trying to be a mom and a wife, and trying to fit more into each day than was humanly possible. Many women overextend themselves, and they do so at their peril. It is an unhealthy way to live, not to mention unrewarding.

Invariably with all this activity and no time to exercise her body, Mary became overweight and unfit. This only made her feel run down and fatigued almost all the time. Instinctively, Mary knew she needed to do something. One day a younger, long-time customer of hers suggested Mary consider water fitness. Mary thought it sounded like fun and probably a more pleasant way to get into shape than having to put up with those embarrassing fitness clubs. The big hurdle was finding a suit and making that first leap of faith into the water. But she had Lisa, the water fitness instructor, who encouraged her and was her womentor.

Lisa worked full time also, but became a certified water fitness instructor to put herself in and around fitness. Lisa was very much committed to her water fitness class and encouraging women to be all they can be. That commitment, her dedication, and her creativity helped make her class very popular and successful. She also had the gift to teach and motivate many people like Mary. Mary finally came and was a hit in the class from the first day. When someone was down, she always had a funny story or something sweet to say to that person. Womentoring became the most natural part of participating in the class for Mary.

Mary absolutely loved working out and helping others have a rewarding time working out. Mary transformed. The weight started coming off and she had energy to do her job and do more with her husband and family. The stronger she got the more she wanted to do. Confident now of her new look and strength, she joined the same fitness club as her husband. It took over a year but she lost 80 pounds and has kept it off. By then everyone just assumed that Mary was a fitness junkie. Mary was so hooked on water fitness she was in the pool practically every day.

At one point, I suggested that Mary become a fitness instructor for my program. That suggestion was like launching a rocket. Mary

> *The great end of life is not knowledge, but action*
> — *Thomas Fuller*

could hardly contain her excitement. She got her own equipment and studied hard with Lisa for the certification. She started coming before and after work to soak up as many ideas as she could for her future classes. In time, Mary passed her certification for teaching water fitness and took over Lisa's class!

Mary's class enrollment had the maximum number of attendees each month. Because she empathizes so well with everyone who comes to her class, many of the women immediately connect with her. They just love being around her and her positive energy. She really knows how to motivate her classes to help them expend the stress that built up during the day at work. Everyone goes home invigorated and happy. Mary has perfected an ongoing personal challenge and a challenge for her classes. I also like Mary's motto that she borrowed from author Christiane Northrup: "Caring for myself is not self indulgence, it is self preservation (and that is an act of political warfare)." I believe women have always been warriors, we just didn't remember it until now.

In the meantime, Lisa started her own business and Mary sold hers and took early retirement. The kids had left home so why was she still working so hard? Her husband was in total support of his new Mary. She was already a pretty person but now she radiated happiness and health with the hint of a jock. There's that new attitude that springs up from the healing properties of water!

MARILYN & RICHARD'S STORY

Marilyn and Richard are a happily married couple in their 50s. They started to come to the pool together after Richard had a terrible skiing accident and required physical therapy. Fortunately, they decided to make water fitness a part of Richard's therapy. They are the first to assert that water fitness has changed both their lives.

Richard is the skiing coach for the local high school ski team and he never misses a competition. An injury because of skiing could be traumatic for anyone as committed to the sport as Richard, but he is a strong man, physically and mentally. He is definitely not the type to feel sorry for himself. Instead, he is very determined to regain his strength in the water so he can walk again. There is no doubt that he has every intention of skiing again. I admire his courage and I applaud him for his in-

174

dependent spirit, working with his wheel chair and not against it.

I have learned much from Richard. He has given me very good insight on improvements for

They are able who think they are able

— Virgil

accessibility between the parking lot and the edge of the pool. He loves the accessibility bay that allows him to let himself in the deep water by himself. It has also been very interesting to see him interact with a group of very strong-minded women. He adds to the challenge if anyone starts to wimp out and we do the same for him. When you see him working out as hard as he can despite his physical challenges, he is an inspiration. You can see and admire his determination.

The class Richard attends say they are not competitive, but that just means not with each other. They are very tough on themselves and have come to understand pacing and real exertion. You can sweat in the water, believe me! I think Richard has had some influence on our team spirit. Team spirit is very important to keep individuals motivated and working hard.

As a couple, Marilyn and Richard have always been into fitness and they will continue to make it a regular part of their life with or without a disability. They come three times a week and encourage each other to push harder. Richard always works independently, but within our class. He has improved his posture, limb movement, and strength while listening to my class instructions.

It is interesting, almost amusing to me that Richard has assumed this role that I call "keeper of the gate." He lets the new folks know the scoop as they enter into the water. He always gives extra attention in his super coaching (remember, he's still a high school coach) way to each new person that comes to my class. He knows how much that helps their learning curve and begins to make them part of the team. And I encourage this. This is Richard's attempt to womentor.

It is heartwarming to see how much support Marilyn gives her husband. She is always in the pool with him working out. She has a great positive attitude and I don't think she skipped a beat during his recovery. She always nudges him, but never quite pushing.

Marilyn has noticed a great deal of improvement in her own strength since beginning water exercise. The benefits pay off as she puts in and takes out the wheelchair many times a day. All the new, extra chores such as gardening and chopping wood that have become her job use to increase her neck and shoulder pain, but now they have become routine without increasing fatigue. The breathing exercises from the work that she does in deep water have reconditioned her diaphragm. She notices this because of her stronger voice. She loves to sing and knows this is another good thing that water has helped bring back into her life.

According to Marilyn, Richard is a marvel at his quarterly checkups. His physical therapist is impressed with his consistent, steady improvements. He is always gaining and not losing in his fight to get back to walking on his own again. Marilyn treats him with such respect. There is no question that they are very supportive of each other. It is very refreshing to be around a couple that are as loving to each other. Marilyn and Richard really do uphold the commitment they have to each other even "in sickness and in health." They think healthy, they eat healthy, they see themselves as healthy and so does everyone else. I feel privileged to know them.

176

DJ & JOHN'S STORY

DJ and John also have a very loving relationship like Marilyn and Richard. They are a retired couple in their late 70s and they have always been active and into being healthy. They moved here in the summer of 1990 and found water fitness through their physical therapist. They have been dedicated water fitness participants ever since they participated in their first class. John is one of the main reasons men are comfortable in the class. It only took that first guy to come with his wife that made a difference for all the other guys to come later.

Through two surgeries and numerous medical emergencies, water fitness has remained the one constant in their life. They are sure that without it they would stiffen up, lose range of motion and strength and be in bad shape. They are definitely not in bad shape at all. They even gained the strength and confidence to graduate to the weight room two years ago.

DJ and John are always willing to try things. This sets them apart from so many of their generation because they refuse to get old. Anyway, in preparation for taking their kids and grandbabies to Hawaii, they decided to take a mask, snorkel and fin class last year. Their confidence was heightened when they practiced in their home pool using their own new equipment.

Part of the marvel of these two snorkeling is that DJ doesn't swim and conquered her great fear of water through her success in her water fitness class. She can now put her face in the water and use the snorkel. She uses her Aquajogger to propel through the water and it sure looks like swimming to me! John is just as innovative. He decided to use an Aquajogger so he could stay out longer in the ocean snorkeling!

177

DJ and John both believe like I do that the benefits of a water fitness program go way beyond the exercise alone. They have a relationship with the entire class and the instructor. This class ranges from early 30s to late 80s so age is a non-issue and so is physical ability. The workout level would be considered hard no matter what shape you are in! Brenda, their friend and instructor, keeps them moving and growing stronger. Brenda is a fantastic example of a woman over 60 who works at being in great shape and womentors others by example to follow suit.

What is nice is that you definitely get the feeling that everyone is in this together, and everyone is treated with respect and consideration, ail working together no matter what age or level of fitness. Ultimately, young at heart is the order of the day with them.

John and DJ are world travelers and have led "the good life" and still profess that they have never been associated with people who are more consistently positive, loving and supportive. The social side of belonging to a group where those qualities prevail is beyond measure.

FEY: A LESSON IN PERSISTENCE

Fey is a mature woman in her early 70s and has always had fitness in her life. Deep water fitness has been part of her routine for over 10 years. After she retired, in a very short time her aches and pains turned into crippling arthritis. Not one to let life get her down, she is truly an admirable person; very few people realize the chronic pain she deals with daily. If you watch her walk from the parking lot and down the steps to the pool, you get a sense of the level of pain she must be dealing with. Once you see her in the water you would never know. She is a graceful mermadame who leaves a trail of bubbles in her wake.

Water fitness is the *only* hard exercise that she can do because of the extreme deterioration of her joints. She never misses a class, she always tries the new moves even if her joint won't go that way and she always gets into her target heart rate. There is no doubt in Fey's mind that she would be totally sedentary if it were not for water fitness. These exercises keep her muscles strong and do not add any pain to her joints. And she means that in the most graphic way. Normally, people with chronic pain have 20% less energy than every one else, but Fey does all of her own chores and never misses an opportunity to play with her grandchildren.

> *Let me tell you the secret that has led me to my goal. My strength lies solely in my tenacity*
> — Louis Pasteur

Water classes also help her mentally and emotionally to keep her spirits up as she is so limited in what she can do. She will not be discouraged even though something as simple as walking down the aisle has become more and more difficult. The magical workouts of water fitness help her continue to live joyfully. She is a part of the kindness and courage I am around every day.

DONNA'S STORY

Donna's story is a truly remarkable story that I just love to tell. She is an inspiration. Donna lost 88 pounds and went from a size 26 to a size 14 by *just* doing water fitness classes and no other exercise. She has been taking classes for one year and four months.

Starting with 3 classes a week for about 8 months and then going to 5 a week, Donna really noticed a difference in all aspects of her day to day life. She did not radically change her diet except to be very sensible and attributes all of her weight loss to the exercise alone!

Lots of women talk about losing inches rather than weight because it is not our claim to fame. Gaining strength is our strong point. But it can be done as proven by Donna's dedication. Water made it possible for her to exercise when she could not participate in any other exercise have because of her weight.

She said one of the best things about water for her was that she could work at her own pace, no matter the shape and that no one could see her once she got in the water. Now she wants people to see her in and out of the water.

Water is a great equalizer for so many people. After all, everyone looks the same from the waist or neck up! The water forgives all of our shortcomings, works with what we have and takes us to where we can be.

DIANNE'S STORY

Dianne is my publicist. She is a bright, energetic lady with a marvelous personality. She discovered water fitness while we were working on this book! Dianne has a very special and inspiring story to share.

"For years I struggled with my weight. I have tried every diet you can go on. If you can believe it, I even tried the "one cookie a day" diet! It didn't work either. The worst point in my life was when I had gone on a diet, trying hard to stay with it and actually losing 50 pounds. Well, that was fine, but it did not last. Before long, I not only regained the 50 pounds, but added another 20 pounds on top of that. That's a 70 pound total weight gain after stringent dieting. I was very frustrated.

"About four years ago, my husband's work forced us to move Reno to Los Angeles. This was a big move, since we had lived happily in Reno for over 25 years, raising our children, and making many wonderful friendships.

"Of course, I missed all my friends in Reno. I felt sad and isolated, and most of all I felt fat. And then, as if that were not enough, my feet were numb almost all the time, making it increasingly difficult to walk. What a mess! This was probably one of the lowest points in my life.

"I knew I had to come to terms with myself. The moment had come in my life to completely change who I was and what I stood for. I came to understand that eternity is a single moment and in that moment I was able to grab hold of my life and realize that if I want my life to even come close to the bliss of eternity I must (in the words of a poet William Purty): 'Dance like nobody's watching...', 'Love like you can't be hurt...', 'Sing like nobody's listening...', 'Live like its heaven on earth'.

"The journey first began by getting out of denial. I had to accept the fact that I was fat and not fit. I also could not walk easily. I researched fitness programs and immediately understood that I could not safely start a fitness program alone. So, I visited my physician. I weighed in at 250 pounds and was not healthy in any way: poor nutrition, poor eating habits, and so on.

"I found a private gym with a pool and a private trainer. I interviewed the trainers and learned that these were no dumb jocks. They had degrees in exercise science and knowledge of biomechanics, kinesiology, and human physiology. What really impressed me, however, was their interest and concern about me. It was clear to me from the beginning that anyone working with me would have to assume a joint commitment with me to help in my journey to better health and fitness.

"I started a fitness program that included aerobic and weight training three times a week. As part of my program my trainer and I discussed my eating and nutritional habits. Things definitely needed to change in that department and they did, gradually. No more diets! Diets don't work! Fortunately, I saw changes almost right away as I made responsible choices and the weight started coming off.

"Initially, I was sore from my exercise, but with the support and guidance of my trainer I understood what was happening. None of this was easy, but I felt great. With the support of my family and my trainer, I also came to understand why the food was an issue. This was another significant moment of change and discovery in my life. I was making progress.

"I then made another discovery that would forever change my view of working out. The land-based exercise was fine, and it did help me lose weight and get fit. But there were some definite disadvantages that came with it, like the aches and pains I felt in my joints and my feet. All the while I just accepted this as part of working out. I thought there simply was no other alternative. Then I learned about water fitness. Water fitness was a whole different ball game. The idea of a non-impact workout that could be just as beneficial as a land-based workout was an eye-opener to me.

"I will never forget my experience of putting on my Aquajogger belt for the first time and going in the water. I have never been a big swimmer so I'm glad water fitness does not require swimming. Using the Aquajogger just makes water fitness so easy and so much fun! For my first workout, I started by running in place and trying to remain vertical. I felt so free, I started giggling like a kid. From then on, my workouts in the pool were unlike anything I had every experienced. I just wanted to tell everyone about it. I immediately became an Aquajogger and water fitness fanatic. I not only felt and saw results, but I felt a very distinct overall wellness. There is just something about being in water. It is so calming, yet so invigorating!

"Today I combine a land based workout, with emphasis on weight training, and my regular water fitness workout. I am healthy and fit, I eat a nutritionally balanced diet, and I am happier than I have been in years. My whole attitude towards life has changed. I know that this has even extended over to my personal and professional relationships as well.

"All I went through was worth it, even the not so good parts, because that helped me appreciate all the good things. The process hasn't been easy. But I took baby steps and got to where I am today. You too can reach and stretch yourself as I have. Most of all it takes commitment and knowing you are worth it. This is the most self- caring I have ever been to myself and I feel beautiful – now a smaller egg with stronger legs."

The successes you have read about in this book are just the tip of the proverbial iceberg. Everyone who has made a decision to make water fitness a part of their life has their own unique story to tell. I tried to make a diverse selection, hoping that somehow you would find inspiration from one or two of them. Maybe, if you are already a convert, you may even want to share these stories with other people who you know can benefit from water fitness. At the end of this book I provide details on how you can send in your own personal story. Eventually, we will publish an updated edition of this book and add new stories. So, please write me. I would love to hear your story of success in water.

Chapter 10:
It's a Wonderful Aqua-Life

Today we know that to experience a healthy, balanced, content existence is not something that we can attain simply by changing our diet and exercising. Life is much more than just our body. We must also have peace of mind, we must open ourselves spiritually, and we must have a sense of purpose, of doing something worthwhile with our lives. In a healthy state, all of our life experience encompasses all aspects of our lives and directly involves the lives of others including our loved ones, friends, and the rest of the world. Our aim should be to have wholeness in our lives and in short, that we be at harmony with our minds, bodies, and souls, and beyond. That is what constitutes wholeness.

Ronald E. Kotzsch, Ph.D has some inspiring words about water that says much of what I believe: "Water is the universal solvent. It does effect changes: physical, emotional, mental, and even spiritual. Water can warm or cool us. It can relax or stimulate our emotions and our minds, as well as our bodies. Water can relieve pain, and help heal wounds. It can strengthen our circulation, respiration, and digestive systems. Water can increase our resistance to illness. It can help heal existing illnesses, physical and mental. And water can even induce altered states of consciousness, bringing us to a new and deeper understanding of who we are."

WATER FITNESS FOR WHOLENESS

Water fitness and all this activity involves can be a way to propel you towards wholeness and balance. You may not have started with this as your main goal when you first picked up this book. Perhaps you were hoping to learn a few good workout routines or maybe you just purchased some Aquajogger equipment and wanted to see how you could use it in your own pool. Both are good reasons to begin to enjoy water fitness. I hope I offered you much more. Taking care of yourself, especially in water is a completely different and special way to become fit and healthy. No matter how you turn it, there is just nothing else like it. It's kind of like chocolate. You can scour the earth and you will never find anything even remotely comparable to chocolate. Its beautiful, dark, natural color, its deep, rich, heavenly aroma, its luscious, glorious, creamy taste, and just that nice feeling you get when eating it....

From the moment you enter the pool, water fitness has an effect on you unlike anything else. You are buoyant, and you feel graceful even if out of the water you consider yourself a clumsy oaf. You are caressed and surrounded by a medium that stimulates every nerve in your body. Even if you try to resist, the water makes you feel good. As you stay in the water a little longer, you actually begin to relax. Oh, what a wonderful and marvelous thing water is!

Then you learn some of the breathing and stretching exercises. This is followed by your workouts. You do sit kicks, tire pumps and the rest. You get you heart rate going, and you feel your body. Yes, you actually *feel* your body. It works. Your body is happy and you know it, and so you are happy. There is always that exhilarating feeling once you have done your workout and after you get out of the water. You are always aware of this, at any point during the day as you are out and about, doing whatever you do. You just feel better. And things are easier to do with your newfound strength and stamina and overall well being.

Mind & Soul

Fortunately, there is much more to water fitness then the strictly physical part of it. There is the way water directly affects your frame of mind, your attitude, your awareness of self, and your spiritual side. I believe it is the natural element of water that induces these thoughts and feelings. Water is the catalyst to reconnecting you with your *self*. There is definitely a spiritual element in water.

> *Life shrinks or expands in proportion to our courage*
> — *Anaïs Nin*

The water can help heal you mentally and spiritually. Just overcoming your resistance to water in the first place as a means to become physically fit predisposes you to the other ancillary benefits of the water experience. This is when you begin to understand that to be a water dancer is to be much more than someone who exercises in the water a few times a week. The true water dancer is someone who learns to celebrate life using water as a foundation.

187

To initiate and propel you along, you learn to call on the powers of your mind and spirit to achieve your physical goals. You learn the benefits of visualizations, affirmations, and actualization are part of the process and you are amazed at how effective your mind can be to make dramatic changes in your life. You feel more rested, you have a greater sense of peace, and the anxiety and hypertension you suffered has now dissipated. The powers of the mind really are fantastic. You quickly discover the truth to the concept that "What you think, so you are." The progress you make is very encouraging. Your success eggs you on to further personal achievement. Added to this is your hunger to go within, to explore your spiritual side. Your spirit is definitely a participant in your transformation as you surge towards wholeness. Meditation is a natural outflow of everything else you do as a water dancer.

> *It's not the years in your life but the life in your years that counts*
> – Adlai Stevenson

You begin to realize that meditation can help you still your mind and keep out all the mental "noise" that tends to clutter it. This is a refreshing experience. As you refresh and reinvigorate your body, you are also refreshing and reinvigorating your mind and spirit. Your depth of appreciation for your water fitness program heightens.

Spiritually, you explore other ways to open yourself. Perhaps you try different forms of meditation or relaxation techniques. You experiment with such forms of meditation as Tai Chi, Yoga, or transcendental meditation. You even try aromatherapy, massage, and other ways to pamper yourself. And why not? You instinctively know that emotionally and psychologically this is the way to gain the stability, creativity, and blissful state some call self-actualization or enlightenment. All that you experience makes you want to share this with everyone you know and love. You know you have a very good thing going.

Others

Reaching out to others is the next logical step as you evolve towards wholeness. This can be one of the most rewarding aspects of being a water dancer. This is what makes water fitness so worthwhile to me. I have come to appreciate the benefits of water fitness in and out of the pool.

In the pool, I am so happy to see other people enjoy water, especially adults. For some reason, as children, we have no difficulty expressing our joy of frolicking in water. For most children, going to the pool is a big treat. Playing, swimming, and just having a good time in the water is a fond memory for most of us, but at some point, we "grow up," and the joy of water goes away. This is sad. So when I see grown ups having fun almost like children in the water, it is a comforting sight.

> *The only gift is a portion of thyself*
> — *Ralph Waldo Emerson*

Out of the pool, the benefits are very heart warming as well. From the very beginning, as you make water a part of your life, you have the support of the other people who take the water fitness class. The social atmosphere is very uplifting and encouraging. I use the word *womentoring* to describe how the nurturing side of women is accentuated as women help women get used to the idea of water as a path to wholeness. This woman-to-woman connection is very valuable. This is about the support of female friends, our sisters in life, our fellow mermaids, and it is an important part of our growth as individuals. These are friendships that I see cultivated out of the pool. It is that other dimension of life that gives us wholeness. You will know this is good, because you will feel the happiness of relating to others, of helping and encouraging others. A joy emanates when you do something for yourself and for other people.

At your work and at home, you will notice a difference in your attitude and in the way you treat your family and friends. Other people will notice this, too. It is then that you can begin to truly appreciate the benefits of wholeness and harmony. This is what yields the feeling that your life has value--that what you are doing is worthwhile.

Balance

The concept of balance is very much consistent with the natural properties of water. Michael Odent, author of *Water and Sexuality* writes: "Water constantly tries to recreate a sphere. That is to say a whole, a unity. Water constantly seeks to put together that which is divided. Whether the approach is chemical, physical or symbolic, water always seems to be the mediator, the link, the element that binds things and people together."

Balance in our lives is not an easy achievement, even when we try to do all the right things. As a water dancer, sometimes just getting to the pool is challenge enough. And if you become ill or sidetracked because of travel, this can definitely interfere with your schedule. But no one is perfect. Try not to be too hard on yourself. Strive to better yourself and seek to improve your performance in the pool, but also know that you will have days when you just don't feel quite up to it. Just know that's all right. Know that you will have many more good days for every not so good day.

Freeing yourself from the burden of having to perform consistently all the time will make the water a joy and never drudgery. And this applies to the relationships in your life and how you deal with the world. To reach out should always be a joy. To give of yourself should never be done out of a feeling of obligation. It should always be done freely, and only when you are ready to do it. And sometimes, when dispensing kindness to strangers and the favor goes unappreciated, celebrate the attitude of giving for its own sake. There is definitely a soul gratifying pleasure in such an act. This frees your mind and allows your spirit to soar. Ultimately, you should feel liberated and not constrained in any way. Once you accept this as an acceptable way to make water a part of your life, you really will experience freedom.

In this book, I sought to show you that starting a fitness program that includes water can be one of the most special experiences of your life. In fact, I believe that this book and what I teach can be a pivotal, life changing moment in your life. By living the life of a water dancer, you can transform your mind, body, soul, your relationships, and even your contact with the world around you. Water has done this for me, and I have seen how water has changed the lives of many other people. This to me is true success in life. I also subscribe to Ralph Waldo Emerson's definition of success:

"To laugh often and much; to win the respect of intelligent people and the affection of children; to earn the appreciation of honest critics and endure the betrayal of false friends; to appreciate beauty, to find the best in others; to leave the world a bit better, whether by a healthy child, a garden, or a redeemed social condition; to know even one life has breathed easier because you have lived. This is to have succeeded."

Invitation for Stories

I have always found that the most inspiring things in life are often the stories people share about their unique experiences. This is what reaching out to others is all about. We can learn so much from each other. It is particularly inspiring to hear about people overcoming obstacles in their lives. When it comes to water fitness, sometimes the only way some people gather the courage to get started and the inspiration to keep going are the stories and encouragement they receive from others.

If you have a story you would like to share with me, please write me. I read everything and I plan to put new stories in the next edition of this book.

To contact me, the best thing to do is to write me, care of my publisher at the following address:

Juliana Larson, *Water Dance*
c/o Paper Chase Press
5721 Magazine St., Suite 152
New Orleans, LA 70115

ADDITIONAL RESOURCES TO FURTHER YOUR AQUATIC JOURNEY

Books to Read

Anderson, Bob. *Stretching*. Bolinas, CA: Shelter Publications, 1980.

Angier, Natalie. *Woman: An Intimate Geography*. New York: Houghton Mifflin Company, 1999.

Becker, B., M.D. and Cole, A., M.D. *Comprehensive Aquatic Therapy*. Boston: Butterworth-Heinemann, 1997.

Blach, James and Phyllis. *Nutritional Healing*. Wayne, NJ: Avery Publishing, 1992.

Boyle, W., and Saine, A., N.D. *Naturopathic Hydrotherapy*. East Palestine, OH: Buckeye Press, 1988.

Brown, Dick. *Leap: Coach/Mentor*. New York: Regan Books, 1998 (CD for trainer/client relationship)

Buchman, Dian. *The Complete Book of Water Therapy*. New York: E.P. Dutton, 1979.

Campion, Margaret Reid. *Hydrotherapy: Principles and Practice*. Great Britain: Butterworth and Heinemann, 1997.

Case, LeAnne. *Fitness Aquatics*. Champaign, IL: Human Kinetics, 1997.

Casey, Conrad. *Aqua Dynamics*. National Pool and Spa Institute and the National Fitness Foundation, 1985.

Cayleff, Susan. *Wash and Be Healed*. Philadelphia, PA: Temple University Press, 1987.

Cousins, Norman. *Anatomy of an Illness*. New York: Bantam Books, 1979.

Covey, Stephen. *The Seven Habits of the Highly Successful*. New York NY: Fireside Books, 1990.

Croutier, A. L. *Taking the Waters*. New York: Abbeville Press Publishers, 1992.

Dull, Harold. *Watsu: Freeing the Body in Water*. Middletown, CA: Worldwide Aquatic Bodywork Association, 1997.

Elder, Terri. *Aquatic Fitness*. Winston-Salem, NC: Hunter Textbooks, 1993.

Fahey, Thomas, *Basic Weight Training for Men and Women, 2nd Edition*. Mountain View, CA: Mayfield Publishers, 1994.

Forster, Robert and Huey, Linda. *The Complete Waterpower Workout Book*. New York, NY: Random House, 1993.

Haas, Robert. *Eat to Win and Eat to Succeed*. New York, NY: Signet, 1986.

Haaverland and Saunders. *Swimmer's Guide*. Stuart FL, ALSA Publishing, 1995.

Jackson, Ian, *The Breath Play Approach to Whole Life Fitness*, Garden City, NY: Double Day and Company, 1994.

Katz, Jane, *The New W.E.T. Workout: Water Exercise Techniques to For Strengthening, Toning, and Lifetime fitness*, New York, NY: Facts of File, 1996

Mattes, Aaron. *Active and Assistive Isolated Stretching*. Sarasota FL: Aaron Mattes, 1996.

McArdle, Katch. *Exercise Physiology, Energy, Nutrition and Human Performance, 3rd Edition*. Malvern, PA: Lea & Febiger, 1991.

McNeal, Roxanne. *Aquatic Therapy: Uses and Techniques*. Abingdon, MD: A.T. Services, 1988.

McWaters, Glenn. *Deep Water Exercise for Health and Fitness*. Laguna Beach, CA: Publitec Editions, 1988.

Moor, F.B. *Manual of Hydrotherapy and Massage*. Boise, ID: Pacific Press Publishing Association, 1964.

Northrup, Christiane, M.D. *Women Bodies, Women's Wisdom*. Old Tappan, NJ: Flemming H. Revell, 1987.

Odent, Michael. *Water and Sexuality*. New York: Penguin Press, 1990.

Prudden, Bonnie. *Complete Guide to Pain-Free Living*. New York: Ballantine Books, 1984.

_____. *Pain Erasure*. New York: Ballantine Books, 1977.

Skinner, A.T. *Duffield's Exercise in Water*. London: Baillierer Tindall, 1983.

Sova, Ruth. *Aquatics: The Complete Reference Guide for Aquatic Fitness Professionals*. Boston, MA: Jones and Bartlett Publishers, 1992.

_____.*Water Fitness Over 40*, Champaign, IL: Human Kinetics, 1995.

Troeller, Linda. *Healing Waters*. Paris: Marvel, 1997.

Wilson, Edmund. *Consilience: The Unity of Knowledge..* New York: Random House, 1999.

Places to Contact

To call for pools that have a certified instructor teaching their classes:

American Physical Therapy Association
Aquatic Section
1111 Fairfax Street
Alexandria, VA 22314
(703) 206-7686

Aquatic Exercise Association, Inc.
P.O. Box 1609
Nokomis, FL 34274
(941) 486-8600

The Aquatic Therapy and Rehabilitation Institute
1032 South Spring Street
Port Washington, WI 53074
(414) 284-3633

The Council for National Cooperation in Aquatics
P.O. Box 26268
Indianapolis, IN 46226
(317) 546-5108

Fitness Educators of Older Adults Association
759 Chopin Drive, Suite 1
Sunnyvale, CA 94087
(408) 735-9398

International Swimming Hall of Fame
One Hall of Fame Drive
Fort Lauderdale, FL 33316
(214) 637-6282

Jewish Community Center Association
15 East 26th Street
New York, NY 10010
(212) 532-4949

National Recreation and Park Association
Aquatics Section
650 West Higgins
Hoffman Estates, IL 60195
(847) 843-7529

National Spa and Pool Institute
2111 Eisenhower Avenue
Alexandria, VA 22314
(703) 838-0083

President's Council on Physical Fitness and Sports
701 Pennsylvania Avenue, Suite 250
Washington, DC 20004-2608
(202) 272-3421

Swimming Pool Hotline
Consult this organization with pool problems or questions about aquatic equipment, working out in pools, etc. (900) 446-6075 x820

United States Water Fitness Association
Boynton Beach, FL
(561) 732-9908

World Waterpark Association
P.O. Box 14826
Lanexa, KS 66285-4826
(903) 599-0300

People to Contact

Here are some people you can consult about making a contact near your area to join or start a water fitness program:

Batman, Kathy, Water Fitness Instructor, Seattle, WA, (206) 526-2000 x3147

Cole, Ann, Watsu for Two, Easter Seals Pool, Eugene, OR

Garrett, Gwendolyn, Aquatic Rehabilitation, Smithville, VA

Jones, Freda, Ph.D., Aquatic Circuits, Oklahoma City, OK

Kuledge, Sally, Water Fitness Instructor, Newport Beach, CA, 714-646-5974

Meyer, Ruth, Hydrotherapy for Massage, RIM, Detroit, MI

Norris, Janet, Aquatic Flexercise, Frankfort, IN

Osinski, Alison, PhD, Aquatic Consulting, San Diego, CA

Plano Aquatic Solutions, Plano, TX

Starr, Linda Portland, OR,

(503) 223-6251

Tuhune, Terrell, Senior Water Fitness, Salt Lake City, UT

Vaughn, Stephanie, Splash: aquatic shop, Winchester, VA,

(540) 667-0585

Wolford, Sue, Aquatics, Ketchum, ID

Water Fitness Equipment

Consult the companies listed here for specialized water fitness equipment. They are all good sources.

1-800-SAY-LEAP

If you want a great motivational coaching book, call this number.

Aquatic Trends
649 U.S. Highway One, Suite 14
North Palm Beach, FL 33408
(800) 296-5496

Manufacture a stainless steel poolside Water Workout Station.

Excel Sports Science
450 West Fifth Avenue, Suite 100
Eugene, OR 97401
(800) 484-2454

Makers of Aquajogger, and a variety of water fitness equipment.

Force Fins
715 Kimball Avenue
Santa Barbara, CA 93103
(800) FIN-SWIM

Makers of power water fins.

Hydrophonics
880 Calle Plano, Unit J
Camarillo CA 93012
(800) 794-6626

Waterproof and submersible microphones and pool sound systems.

Hydro-Tone Fitness Systems
16691 Gothard Street, Suite M
Hungtinton Beach CA 92647
(800) 622-8663

Makers of plastic handheld dumbbells and resistive devices.

Polar Monitor
99 Seaview Boulevard
Port Washington NY 11050
(800) 742-4478

Makers of a heart-rate monitor with a chest strap and a wrist telemetry unit. A top-of-the-line model allows you to download to your computer.

Index

warm up: exercise, 87;
   thermal, 87-88
warming down, 87
water fitness: friends, 48;
   footwear, 94; men and,
   155
"water is too easy" (myth),
   28
water: massage, 168;
   therapy, 127; workouts,
   37, 72, 85-86, 138, 161;
   webbed gloves, 94;
   women and, 58;
   transforming effects of, 51
water workout: regular, 24,
31, 46, 77, 138, 148, 154
well-being, 19, 123, 157, 187
wheel chair bound, 126
Williams, Esther, 62
women: as swimmers, 61;
   intuition, 54; pregnant,
   138
womentoring, 49, 51-52, 173
words: power of, 70
workaholics, 50

Y
YMCA, 31, 126, 151
Yoga, 189
"You are what you think.,"
69

Z
Ziegler, Erica, 138

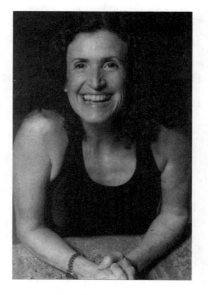

ABOUT THE AUTHOR

Juliana Larson, as author, lecturer, and certified fitness instructor, writes and speaks worldwide on the topics of water fitness and wellness for women. Larson is also a member of numerous water fitness and health organizations, including the Aquatic Exercise Association (AEA), United States Water Fitness Association (USWFA), and the National Arthritis Foundation. Larson is also the recipient of the prestigious USWFA Glenn McWaters Excellence Award in recognition for her work in deep water aqua fitness instruction.

Larson's consulting company, Aquatic Solutions, provides aquatic training and certification, hydrotherapy/massage business management, and personal programs for both the physically fit and physically challenged. Larson has authored numerous articles on the subject of wellness and water fitness for a variety of trade and commercial publications, and has co-written and produced two videos: "Bouncebackability" and "The Complete Aquajogger Water Fitness Workout."

Juliana Larson lives in Eugene, Oregon with her husband.

Other books from Paper Chase Press

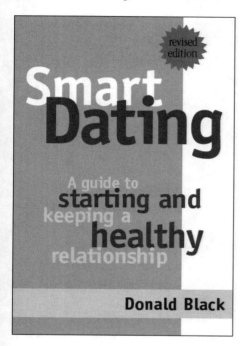

Smart Dating: Starting and Keeping a Healthy Relationship
Donald Black
paperback, 256 pages

Donald Black, bestselling author and creator of the successful *Smart Dating* workshops, has guided thousands through the sometimes challenging world of dating and relationships.

"Black doesn't believe games, tricks, or formulas lead to perfect relationships... He gives you the principles that work and points in the right direction."
-Tucson Citizen

"*Smart Dating* is a book every single person should keep on their night stand."
-The Norman Transcript

"*Smart Dating* is straightforward and easy-to-read... definitely will work to your advantage."
-Hugh B. Jones, President,
Southeast Singles Assoc.

$14.95

Other books from Paper Chase Press

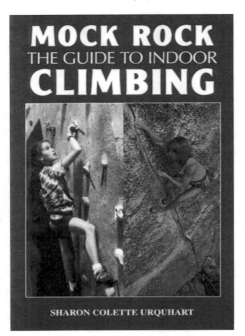

Mock Rock: The Guide to Indoor Climbing
Sharon Colette Urquhart
paperback, 124 pages

Have you ever wondered what it was like to climb a sheer rock face, but were afraid to try? Indoor climbing is a good place to start, and this book helps you get off the ground.

> "Indoor Climbing is the fastest growing sport in the country today. This is an informative book for those who are curious about climbing or for those who are ready to delve into this exciting sport - it should be your first piece of climbing equipment."
> -Hans Florine, Professional climber,
> *'91 World Champion speed climbing*

> "Superb! An easy to use and fun to read introduction to climbing"
> -Sam Davidson,
> *The Access Fund*

$12.95

Other books from Paper Chase Press

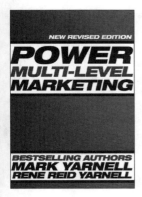

Power Multi-Level Marketing:
Building from ground zero to a global network
Mark Yarnell, Rene Reid Yarnell
paperback, 224 pages

This is an excellent start from ground zero, step by step instruction to the world of MLM. Learn how to select the right company for you, the basics of recruiting, presentations, training and support, and solid tips on how to succeed. If you follow this book, you can duplicate the success of the Yarnells to build a global network.

"*Power Multi-Level Marketing* effectively conveys both advice and inspiration to newcomers to network marketing."
-Howard Rothman,
Amazon.com Non-fiction editor

"This is essential reading for all serious network marketers. A must buy for seasoned veterans as well as those just getting started."
-Spencer Montague,
NuSkin International

$14.95

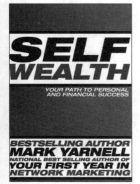

Self Wealth: Your Path to Personal & Financial Success
Mark Yarnell
hardcover, 240 pages

"*Self-Wealth* is one of the best personal and financial achievement books I've read in years!"
-Scott DeGarmo, Publisher,
Success Magazine

$21.95

AquaJogger®
Water Fitness Products

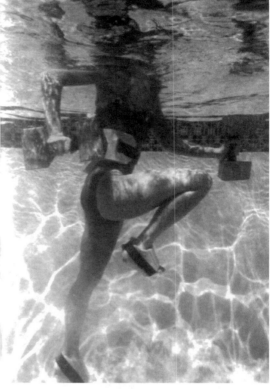

AquaJogger Water Fitness Products have been taking the impact out of exercise and fitness programs since 1987 when its patented buoyancy belt was introduced. This unique flotation device quickly captured the attention and the imagination of fitness and sports medicine professionals around the world. It wasn't long until land based aerobics programs began moving into the forgiving environment of water and a new fitness industry was born. AquaJogger continues to lead the way in this awakening industry with a full line of water fitness products.
For more information:

AquaJogger Water Fitness Products

p.o. box 1453
Eugene, Oregon 97440
tel. **800.922.9544** or **541.484.2454**
fax. **541.484.0501**
e-mail. **info@aquajogger.com**
www.aquajogger.com

Order AquaJogger® Products:

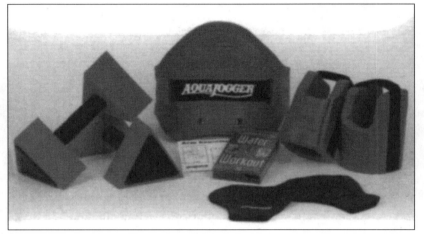

Water Fitness System

AquaJogger's complete system is now available in blue and purple. Includes Buoyancy Belt, AquaRunners®, DeltaBells®, Webbed Pro Gloves, and Video Tape.

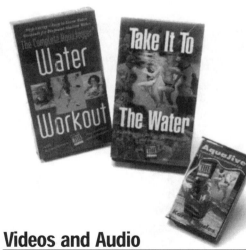

Videos and Audio

The Complete AquaJogger Water Workout
1 hour video featuring 60 different exercises and the latest techniques. Beginners through advanced.

Take it to the Water
1 hour water running video for sports conditioning and recovery.

AquaJive audio cassette
30 minutes of workout music and poolside instruction.

To order Paper Chase Press books,

call 1-800-864-7991, or fill out the form:

Please send me _____ copy(ies) of *Smart Dating*, paperback

Please send me _____ copy(ies) of *Mock Rock*, paperback

Please send me _____ copy(ies) of *Power Multi-Level Marketing*, paperback

Please send me _____ copy(ies) of *Self Wealth*, hardcover

Name _____

Address _____

_____

_____

_____

Signature (for credit card purchases) _____

Please indicate credit card: Visa _____   MC _____

Credit card number _____ expires _____

Fill out form and send a check or money order in US funds only.

All payments made to: PAPER CHASE PRESS.

Send to: Paper Chase Press, 5721 Magazine St., Suite 152, New Orleans LA 70115

Add $5.00 S&H for each book ordered in the US (call for outside of US).

Allow up to 4 weeks for delivery.